I0702017

Table of Contents

INTRODUCTION

Interested in cutting meat out of your diet, but not fish? Or are you considering going vegetarian but want some protein options beyond plants?

Looking for a healthier diet? The benefits of being a pescatarian might get you hooked.

Pescatarians have a lot in common with vegetarians. They eat fruits, veggies, nuts, seeds, whole grains, beans, eggs, and dairy, and stay away from meat and poultry. But there's one way they part company from vegetarians: Pescatarians eat fish and other seafood.

Consider the pescatarian diet. This plan more like a lifestyle is vegetarian with one key difference: You also eat fish and seafood.

A pescatarian is someone who adds fish and seafood to a vegetarian diet. Some pescatarians may eat eggs and dairy, while others may not.

There are many reasons people choose to forgo red meat and poultry, but still eat fish.

Some people choose to add fish to a vegetarian diet so they can get the health benefits of a plant-based diet plus heart-healthy fish.

Others might be trying to curb the environmental impact of their diet. For some, it might be simply a matter of taste.

This book looks more about the benefits and drawbacks of a pescatarian diet, including exactly what a pescatarian does and doesn't eat.

WHAT IS A PESCATARIAN?

Most simply, a pescatarian is someone who doesn't eat red meat or poultry, but does eat fish and other seafood.

The term pescatarian was coined in the early 1990s and is a combination of the Italian word for fish, "pesce," and the word "vegetarian." Sometimes it's spelled "pescetarian," but this means the same thing.

In scientific literature, this diet is often described as "pesco-vegetarian," and is lumped into the spectrum of vegetarianism.

By that definition, a pescatarian is someone who chooses to eat a vegetarian diet, but who also eats fish and other seafood.

It's a largely plant-based diet of whole grains, nuts, legumes, produce and healthy fats, with seafood playing a key role as a main protein source.

9

Many pescatarians also eat dairy and eggs.

Of course, just as vegetarian diets can vary widely, so can pescatarian ones. It's possible to eat a meat-free diet that's full of processed starches, junk food and fish sticks, rather than a healthier one based on whole foods.

A pescatarian is someone who follows a mostly vegetarian diet but also eats fish and seafood.

WHY DO PEOPLE CHOOSE A PESCATARIAN DIET?

There are several reasons people may choose to eat a pescatarian diet. Here are some of the main ones.

Health Benefits

There are many proven benefits to plant-based diets, including a lower risk of obesity and chronic diseases like heart disease and diabetes.

According to research, you can get many of those protective benefits from a pescatarian diet too.

One study found that women who were pescatarians gained 2.5 fewer pounds (1.1 kg) each year than women who ate meat.

And people who shifted their diet in a more plant-based direction gained the least amount of weight, showing that reducing your animal consumption may be good for you no matter your current eating patterns.

Another study concluded that pescatarians had a lower risk of developing diabetes at 4.8%, compared to omnivores at 7.6%.

Additionally, one large study looked at people who ate meat rarely or were pescatarians. They had a 22% lower risk of dying from heart disease compared to regular meat-eaters.

ENVIRONMENTAL CONCERNS

Raising livestock comes with a high environmental cost.

According to the United Nations, raising livestock contributes to 15% of all human-made carbon emissions.

In contrast, producing fish and seafood has a lower carbon footprint than producing any type of animal meat or cheese.

A 2014 study calculated that diets of fish eaters caused 46% less greenhouse gas emissions than the diets of people who ate at least a serving of meat a day .

ETHICAL REASONS

11

Ethics can be a major reason why people choose to go vegetarian. It can be a major reason for pescatarians too.

Some of the ethical reasons people choose not to eat meat include:

- Opposing slaughter: They don't want to kill animals for food.
- Inhumane factory practices: They refuse to support factory farms that raise livestock in inhumane conditions.
- Poor labor conditions: They refuse to support factory farms that have poor conditions for their workers.
- Humanitarian reasons: They consider producing grain for animal feed an unjust use of land and resources when there's so much hunger in the world.

Eliminating land animals from your diet addresses some of these ethical concerns. That said, aquaculture and overfishing can also be problematic.

Monterey Bay Aquarium's Seafood Watch program is an excellent resource for finding fish that are caught or farmed in ethical ways.

There are several reasons people choose a pescatarian diet, including concerns about health, ethics and the environment.

WHAT DO PESCATARIANS EAT?

A typical pescatarian diet is primarily vegetarian with the addition of seafood.

Pescatarians Do Eat

- Whole grains and grain products
- Legumes and their products, including beans, lentils, tofu and hummus
- Nuts and nut butters, peanuts and seeds
- Seeds, including hemp, chia and flaxseeds
- Dairy, including yogurt, milk and cheese
- Fruits
- Vegetables
- Fish and shellfish
- Eggs

Pescatarians Don't Eat

- Beef

- Chicken

- Pork

- Lamb

- Turkey

- Wild game

A healthy pescatarian diet is largely made up of minimally processed plant foods, plus seafood and possibly dairy and eggs.

BENEFITS OF ADDING FISH TO A VEGETARIAN DIET

There are many health benefits of adding fish to a vegetarian diet.

Many people are concerned that completely excluding animal products or avoiding animal flesh could lead to a low intake of certain key nutrients.

In particular, vitamins B12, zinc, calcium and protein can be somewhat harder to get on a vegan diet.

Adding seafood, including fish, crustaceans and mollusks, to a vegetarian diet can provide beneficial nutrients and variety.

Get More Omega-3s

Fish is the best way to get omega-3 fatty acids.

Some plant foods, including walnuts and flaxseeds, contain alpha-linolenic acid (ALA), a type of omega-3 fat. However, this type of ALA is not easily converted to eicosapentaenoic acid (EPA) and docosahexaenoic acid (DHA) in the body.

DHA and EPA have additional health benefits, helping not just the heart, but also brain function and mood.

In contrast, oily fish, such as salmon and sardines, contains EPA and DHA.

Boost Your Protein Intake

Humans only need about 0.8 grams of protein per 2.2 pounds (1 kg) of body weight daily to stay healthy. That's about 54 grams for a 150-pound (68-kg) person.

However, many people prefer to eat more protein than that.

A high-protein diet can be hard to achieve with just plant proteins, especially if you don't want extra carbs or fat with your protein.

Fish and other seafood offer an excellent source of lean protein.

Seafood Is Packed With Other Nutrients

Beyond omega-3s and protein, seafood is rich in several other nutrients.

For instance, oysters are extremely high in vitamin B12, zinc and selenium. Just one oyster delivers 133% of the RDI for vitamin B12 and 55% of the RDI for zinc and selenium.

Mussels are also super rich in vitamin B12 and selenium, as well as manganese and the rest of the B vitamins.

White fish varieties such as cod and flounder don't deliver much omega-3 fats, but they are a source of extremely lean protein.

For example, just 3 ounces of cod provide 19 grams of protein and less than a gram of fat. Cod is also an excellent source of selenium and a good source of phosphorus, niacin and vitamins B6 and B12.

You'll Have Extra Options

Being a vegetarian can be limiting at times.

Eating out at restaurants often leaves you with a not-so-healthy choice, with dishes like cheesy pasta as the main "veggie" option.

If health at least partially motivates your food choices, then becoming pescatarian will give you more options.

And fish is generally a good one, especially if you get it baked, grilled or sautéed, as opposed to deep-fried (21Trusted Source).

Adding seafood to a vegetarian diet gives you more options and is a good way to get protein, omega-3s and other nutrients.

PESCATARIAN DIET FOR WEIGHT LOSS

Is a pescatarian diet good for weight loss? It just might be. A 2022 review in the International Journal of Environmental Research and Public Health suggests that vegetarians tend to eat significantly fewer calories each day than their meat-eating counterparts. Plus, all the fiber in plant-based eating helps keep us full, which means we don't feel as hungry in between meals.

To promote a healthy weight loss of 1 to 2 pounds a week, we set this plan at 1,200 calories a day and included modifications to bump up the calories to 1,500 or 2,000 calories a day, depending on your needs.

IS THE PESCATARIAN DIET RIGHT FOR YOU?

17

Trying to go plant-based with your diet, but don't want to give up fish? You've come to the right place. Enter the pescatarian diet (also called pesco-vegetarian), which is very similar to the popular Mediterranean diet.

Pesce is the Italian word for fish. In addition to fruits, vegetables, whole grains, legumes, eggs and dairy products, pescatarians also eat fish and shell fish. Here's your ultimate guide to pescatarian eating.

What You Can Eat

Those following the pescatarian diet can eat a wide range of foods that contribute to a balanced macronutrient profile and provide the vitamins and minerals needed for optimal health.

✓ Seafood

The seafood on the pescatarian diet may include freshwater fish such as trout or perch, saltwater fish like salmon or tuna, and shellfish including shrimp, oysters, clams, and more.

✓ Dairy Foods and Eggs

Most pescatarians eat eggs and dairy (such as cheese, yogurt, and milk), although some do not. Technically, a pescatarian who eats eggs and dairy would be called a lacto-ovo-pescatarian.

✓ Fruits and Vegetables

There are no limits on the types of fruits and vegetables included in this eating plan. Eat the rainbow, and fill up on produce to receive the full health benefits; add dark leafy greens, bright red, yellow, and orange peppers, eggplant, corn, blueberries, kiwi, and other fruits and veggies.

✓ Beans and Legumes

Beans and legumes are an excellent addition to the pescatarian diet because they are rich sources of plant-based protein.

✓ Nuts and Seeds

Nuts and seeds are a great addition to the pescatarian diet because they are rich sources of healthy fats. Excellent choices include walnuts, almonds, sunflower seeds, and chia seeds.

✓ Grains

Pescatarians can eat a wide range of grains, including wheat, corn, barley, rye, rice, oats and others. People with celiac disease or those avoiding gluten also avoid gluten on the pescatarian diet.

✓ Oils

Those who follow the pescatarian diet can use a wide variety of oils in their cooking and seasoning of food.

Some common examples are olive oil, sesame oil, walnut oil, and canola oil. Many types of oil are good sources of monounsaturated and polyunsaturated fats, which contribute to cardiovascular health.

What You Cannot Eat

There is only one class of foods that those who eat a pescatarian diet do not eat: meats. Regardless of whether or not you eat certain animal products like yogurt or cheese, if you follow the pescatarian diet, you won't eat meat or meat products. That means you'll not only avoid red meat (like beef or bison), but you'll also avoid poultry, lamb, pork, and game (such as venison).

HOW TO PREPARE THE PESCATARIAN DIET & TIPS

The pescatarian diet is a lifestyle. If you decide to eat a pescatarian diet, you can eat meals and snacks whenever you'd like, with no specific recommendations or restrictions on portion size.

The pescatarian diet is likely safe and probably beneficial if you have a health condition such as diabetes, celiac disease, or heart disease. But you should always check with a healthcare provider first and ensure you're getting the right mix of nutrients for your body.

If you are pregnant, avoid raw fish (e.g., sushi and sashimi) and watch out for the mercury levels in the fish you eat.3 You'll also want to be cautious about mercury if you are breastfeeding or have small children who eat pescatarian too. Fish high in mercury include swordfish, shark, some types of mackerel, marlin, and some types of tuna. Talk to a healthcare provider such as a physician or registered dietitian for help if you are unsure what to eat.

What to Eat

- Seafood
- Fruits and vegetables
- Grains
- Dairy products and eggs

What Not to Eat

- Red meat
- Poultry
- Pork
- Wild game

Pros of the Pescatarian Diet

- May Protect from Disease: Some studies have shown that pescatarians have a lower risk of diseases such as diabetes, high blood pressure, and metabolic disorders that increase the risk of heart attacks and stroke.

- May Be Easier to Follow Than Vegetarianism: Some people who choose to eliminate meat from their diets may find that following a pescatarian diet is more manageable than following a strictly vegetarian diet because it is easier to get enough protein each day with the addition of seafood.

- May Promote Healthy Weight: When you replace meat-based meals with plant-based meals, you are likely to cut calories and fat from your diet to help you reach and maintain a healthy weight.

- Can Benefit the Environment: Some people follow a pescatarian diet because of the positive impact certain sustainable seafood choices can have on the environment. Raising and processing meat takes up land and contributes to dangerous emissions. By reducing our dependency on meat and making sustainable fish choices, we do our part to help create a healthier planet.

To feel better about your impact on the environment, use the information provided by The Monterey Bay Aquarium Seafood Watch to find responsibly sourced seafood. Enter the name of the fish you prefer and get specific recommendations for buying the best fish.

There is even an app that you can use when you're shopping.

Cons of the Pescatarian Diet

While the pescatarian diet has a lot of advantages, there are also a couple of disadvantages.

- Some Seafood Is High In Mercury: All seafood and shellfish have some mercury content, and certain fish have a higher concentration than others. When you eat fish, mercury is absorbed through digestion and enters the bloodstream, traveling to every organ in your body. It can cross the blood-brain barrier and , in excess, it can cause damage to your central nervous system.
- Groceries Can Be Costly: Buying the primary foods of this eating plan (fruits, vegetables, and fresh fish) can be expensive. But you don't always have to buy fresh—many bulk bags of frozen fruits and vegetables are just as healthy as the fresh versions. Canned fish is economical and easy to store.

IS THE PESCATARIAN DIET A HEALTHY CHOICE FOR YOU?

Current guidelines set forth by the Department of Agriculture (USDA) suggest filling your plate with a balanced mix of protein (which could be from meat, fish, or plant-based sources), grains, fruits, vegetables, and dairy.8 The pescatarian diet meets that standard when meals are balanced with USDA-recommended foods and nutrients.

There's no official calorie count for the pescatarian diet, which means no need for calorie counting. The number of calories you need will vary based on your goals (weight loss, weight maintenance, or weight gain), age, weight, sex, and activity level).9 Use this calculator to determine the right calorie goal for you.

IS THE PESCATARIAN DIET RIGHT FOR YOU?

A pescatarian diet is a good option for anyone who wants to focus on a more plant-based diet but doesn't want to become a full vegetarian or vegan. Eating a pescatarian diet allows more flexibility because you can continue to incorporate animal protein from seafood.

HOW TO MAKE THE SWITCH TO A PESCATARIAN DIET

Since the pescatarian diet continues to allow eggs, milk products and seafood, the switch shouldn't be too hard. But if you feel overwhelmed, just start small.

- Start by eliminating red meat.
- Try incorporating a "Meatless Monday" and slowly transition over to eliminate all animal protein except seafood.
- Include a wide variety of food, especially plant-based protein sources such as beans, lentils, tofu, nuts and seeds. (In other words, don't eat fish three times a day, seven days a week as your only protein source.)

Overall, a pescatarian diet offers many health benefits. If you would like to follow a more plant-based diet but still retain some flexibility, it might be a great option for you. Your primary care doctor can help you figure out what kind of diet is right for your health goals.

PESCATARIAN VS. MEDITERRANEAN DIET: WHICH IS HEALTHIER?

The pescatarian lifestyle and the Mediterranean diet share some similarities. Both plans focus on fruits, vegetables and whole grains. But on the Mediterranean diet, you:

- Eat meat: You can have any type of meat on the Mediterranean diet, but should minimize red and processed meats.
- Emphasize olive oil: Both diets allow olive oil, but it's a key component of the Mediterranean diet.
- Eat less dairy: The Mediterranean diet typically includes only a few servings of dairy each week.

"Following the Mediterranean diet is a proven way to lower your risk of heart disease," Execpt says. "But studies also show you can get similar results with the pescatarian diet. An important key with either diet is to choose whole foods over processed foods as much as possible."

Choose what works for you

Following a pescatarian diet can improve your health but it's not for everyone. "Some people really enjoy lean chicken, or they don't like fish," notes Execpt. "In these cases, going pescatarian probably isn't a good idea. Consider the Mediterranean diet instead. The best diet for you is the most nutrient-filled one you can stick to long term."

Drawbacks of a Pescatarian Diet

As with many things in life, you can sometimes have too much of a good thing. Fish and seafood are no exception. For instance, some types of fish, like tuna, swordfish, and tilefish, have moderate to high levels of mercury.

Mercury is a heavy metal that can cause health problems, especially for babies and children. That's why the government recommends that young children, along with women of childbearing age or who are pregnant or breastfeeding, mostly eat fish that's low in mercury. If you go pescatarian, consider choosing lower-mercury types of fish, like salmon, mackerel, herring, sardines, and lake trout.

Getting rid of red meat from your diet may rob you of iron, especially if you're a woman who's menstruating. You can get iron from other sources, like dark leafy greens, tofu, and lentils. Manufacturers also add it to some foods, like cereal. But it's always good to talk to your doctor before starting a new diet to make sure you cover all your nutritional bases.

Keep in mind that food that's labeled "meat-free" or "vegetarian" isn't automatically healthy. It can still be high in sugar and fat, especially if it's processed. That's why eating unprocessed foods as often as possible is

the best way to go -- no matter what type of diet you
follow.

There can be some drawbacks to eating a pescatarian
diet. It's easy to overeat carbs and some fish are high in
mercury.

WHICH NUTRIENTS MAY BE LACKING IN A PESCATARIAN DIET?

Like all diets, a pescatarian diet needs to be balanced
and varied in order to be healthy. The lack of red meat
means iron intakes could be sub-optimal. It is therefore
important to include plant-based sources of iron, such
as spinach and broccoli, and opt for low-sugar breakfast
cereals, as these are fortified with vitamins and
minerals.

Some pescatarians do not consume eggs or dairy, which
can mean they may be lacking in essential nutrients
such as calcium, phosphorus, vitamin B12 and zinc.
Therefore, if you are planning to embark on this dietary
change, it is important to ensure you eat a healthy,
balanced diet and that it provides all the nutrition you
need.

SHOULD I BE WORRIED ABOUT MERCURY LEVELS IN FISH?

All fish contain varying amounts of mercury a pollutant that can be highly toxic to our nervous system. We're all advised to include at least two portions of fish per week, with at least one being an oily variety such as salmon – a portion is 140g (cooked weight).

However, for certain types of fish, there are recommendations for the maximum you should eat, too. In this regard, the NHS advises that the general population eat no more than four portions of oily fish per week. Women who are planning to conceive or are pregnant or breastfeeding are advised to eat no more than two portions of oily fish per week, as mercury can affect the nervous system and may cause development delays in infants exposed to it in the womb.

Shark, swordfish and marlin contain concentrated sources of mercury, so it is recommended that they should be avoided by women who are planning to conceive or are pregnant or breastfeeding, and by all children.

You can safely eat as many portions of white fish per week as you like, except for the following, which may contain similar levels of pollutants as oily fish:

- Sea bream
- Sea bass
- Turbot
- Halibut

- Rock salmon (also known as dog fish)

As a pescatarian, you're likely to eat a lot of fish, so be aware that these five fish and brown meat from crab shouldn't be eaten too often.

1-DAY MEAL PLAN

Here, we give examples of recipes for meals that a person might consider when choosing a pescatarian diet:

Breakfast

Sardines on crostini

Sardines are an excellent source of omega-3s. Using spinach to make a pesto spread on the crostini provides a source of vitamin C and vitamin A. The vitamin C helps increase the amount of iron a person absorbs.

This recipe uses canned sardines, but it is also possible to use fresh sardines or anchovies. Starting the day with protein increases the feeling of fullness, and the pesto adds healthful greens that are a source of iron.

Lunch

Classic baked falafel

Tahini is good source of plant protein and omega-3s. Chickpeas are also a good source of plant protein and fiber. Add a healthful Mediterranean salad to this recipe to create a filling lunch.

Dinner

Roasted salmon with shallot grapefruit sauce

Salmon provides omega-3s essential fatty acids.

Strong-flavored fish go very well with citrus fruits such as grapefruit. The addition of grapefruit to this recipe also adds vitamin C and fiber, and it counts toward the 2 servings of fruit that a person should eat per day.

Most pescatarians only have seafood once a day or a few times a week, not multiple times per day. Another option for a one-day meal plan could be:

- Breakfast: Oatmeal made with coconut milk topped with fresh berries, chia seeds, and almond butter
- Lunch: A grain bowl made with quinoa, sweet potatoes, kale, and chickpeas.
- Dinner: Grilled salmon and lemony asparagus served with a baked potato and a side salad

7-DAY PESCATARIAN DIET PLAN

This pescatarian diet meal plan combines healthy plant-based ingredients with tasty fish and seafood for a flavor-packed, nutritious week.

Day 1

Breakfast (290 calories)

- 1 serving Strawberry-Pineapple Smoothie
- 1 clementine

A.M. Snack (97 calories)

- 1/2 cup nonfat plain Greek yogurt
- 1/2 cup blackberries

Lunch (366 calories)

- 1 serving Vegetarian Niçoise Salad

P.M. Snack (64 calories)

- 1 cup raspberries

Dinner (395 calories)

- 1 serving Roasted Salmon Caprese
- 1 serving Basic Quinoa

Daily Totals: 1,213 calories, 63 g protein, 119 g carbohydrates, 30 g fiber, 57 g fat, 1,273 mg sodium

To make it 1,500 calories: Add 1 cup nonfat plain Greek yogurt and 20 unsalted dry-roasted almonds to P.M. snack.

To make it 2,000 calories: Include all additions for the 1,500-calorie day, plus add 1 whole-wheat English muffin with 2 Tbsp. natural peanut butter to breakfast and add 1 large pear to lunch.

Day 2

Breakfast (278 calories)

- 1 cup nonfat plain Greek yogurt
- 1 serving Maple Granola

A.M. Snack (62 calories)

- 1 medium orange

Lunch (365 calories)

- 1 serving Green Goddess Quinoa Bowls with Arugula & Shrimp
- 1 large pear

P.M. Snack (37 calories)

- 1 medium bell pepper, sliced

Dinner (468 calories)

- 1 serving Cheesy Spinach-&-Artichoke Stuffed Spaghetti Squash

- 2 cups mixed greens
- 1/2 avocado, sliced
- 2 Tbsp. Citrus-Lime Vinaigrette

Daily Totals: 1,209 calories, 57 g protein, 149 g carbohydrates, 37 g fiber, 50 g fat, 937 mg sodium

To make it 1,500 calories: Add 1/3 cup unsalted dry-roasted almonds to A.M. snack.

To make it 2,000 calories: Include the addition for the 1,500-calorie day, plus add 1 slice whole-wheat toast with 1 Tbsp. natural peanut butter to breakfast, increase to 2 bell peppers and add 1/3 cup hummus to P.M. snack, and increase to 1 whole avocado at dinner.

Day 3

Breakfast (247 calories)

- 1 serving Parmesan & Vegetable Muffin-Tin Omelets
- 1/2 cup raspberries

A.M. Snack (62 calories)

- 1 medium orange

Lunch (365 calories)

- 1 serving Green Goddess Quinoa Bowls with Arugula & Shrimp
- 1 large pear

P.M. Snack (116 calories)

- 1 large apple

Dinner (421 calories)

- 1 serving Spicy Shrimp Tacos

Daily Totals: 1,210 calories, 53 g protein, 158 g carbohydrates, 32 g fiber, 47 g fat, 1,506 mg sodium

To make it 1,500 calories: Add 22 walnut halves to A.M. snack.

To make it 2,000 calories: Include the addition for the 1,500-calorie day, plus add 1/3 cup unsalted dry-roasted almonds to P.M. snack and add 1 serving Guacamole Chopped Salad to dinner.

Day 4

Breakfast (278 calories)

- 1 cup nonfat plain Greek yogurt
- 1 serving Maple Granola

A.M. Snack (77 calories)

- 1 small apple

Lunch (365 calories)

- 1 serving Green Goddess Quinoa Bowls with Arugula & Shrimp

- 1 large pear

P.M. Snack (62 calories)

- 1 medium orange

Dinner (429 calories)

- 1 serving Curried Sweet Potato & Peanut Soup
- 2 cups mixed greens
- 2 Tbsp. Citrus-Lime Vinaigrette

Daily Totals: 1,211 calories, 57 g protein, 168 g carbohydrates, 31 g fiber, 43 g fat, 992 mg sodium

To make it 1,500 calories: Add 1 medium peach to breakfast and add 2 Tbsp. natural peanut butter to A.M. snack.

To make it 2,000 calories: Include all additions for the 1,500-calorie day, plus add 15 walnut halves to P.M. snack and add 1 whole avocado (sliced) to dinner.

Day 5

Breakfast (247 calories)

- 1 serving Parmesan & Vegetable Muffin-Tin Omelets
- 1/2 cup raspberries

A.M. Snack (66 calories)

- 1/2 cup nonfat plain Greek yogurt

Lunch (365 calories)

- 1 serving Green Goddess Quinoa Bowls with Arugula & Shrimp
- 1 large pear

P.M. Snack (62 calories)

- 1 medium orange

Dinner (478 calories)

- 1 serving Vegetarian Enchilada Casserole
- 1 serving Jason Mraz's Guacamole

Daily Totals: 1,218 calories, 59 g protein, 144 g carbohydrates, 33 g fiber, 51 g fat, 1,182 mg sodium

Meal-prep note: Refrigerate 2 servings of the Vegetarian Enchilada Casserole to have for lunches on Day 6 and Day 7.

To make it 1,500 calories: Add 1/3 cup unsalted dry-roasted almonds to P.M. snack.

To make it 2,000 calories: Include the addition for the 1,500-calorie day, plus add 1 whole-wheat English muffin with 2 Tbsp. natural peanut butter to breakfast and add 1 serving Maple Granola to A.M. snack.

Day 6

Breakfast (255 calories)

- 1 serving Strawberry-Pineapple Smoothie

A.M. Snack (101 calories)

- 1 medium pear

Lunch (357 calories)

- 1 serving Vegetarian Enchilada Casserole

P.M. Snack (78 calories)

- 1 large hard-boiled egg
- Pinch of salt and pepper

Dinner (406 calories)

- 1 serving Baked Halibut with Brussels Sprouts & Quinoa

Daily Totals: 1,198 calories, 56 g protein, 145 g carbohydrates, 31 g fiber, 51 g fat, 1,406 mg sodium

To make it 1,500 calories: Add 1 medium orange to P.M. snack and add 1 serving Guacamole Chopped Salad to dinner.

To make it 2,000 calories: Include all additions for the 1,500-calorie day, plus add 1 whole-wheat English muffin with 2 Tbsp. natural peanut butter to breakfast and add 18 unsalted dry-roasted almonds to A.M. snack.

Day 7

Breakfast (247 calories)

- 1 serving Parmesan & Vegetable Muffin-Tin Omelets
- 1/2 cup raspberries

A.M. Snack (131 calories)

- 1 large pear

Lunch (357 calories)

- 1 serving Vegetarian Enchilada Casserole

P.M. Snack (16 calories)

- 1 cup sliced cucumber
- Pinch of salt and pepper

Dinner (466 calories)

- 1 serving Coconut-Curry Cod Stew with Sweet Potato & Rice
- 2 cups mixed greens
- 2 Tbsp. Citrus-Lime Vinaigrette

Daily Totals: 1,218 calories, 52 g protein, 148 g carbohydrates, 30 g fiber, 51 g fat, 1,567 mg sodium

To make it 1,500 calories: Add 1 slice whole-wheat bread with 1 Tbsp. natural peanut butter to breakfast and add 1/4 cup hummus to P.M. snack.

To make it 2,000 calories: Include all additions for the 1,500-calorie day, plus add 22 unsalted dry-roasted almonds to A.M. snack and add 1 whole avocado (sliced) to dinner.

SAMPLE SHOPPING LIST

If you buy fresh fish, it usually needs to be cooked or frozen within a few days of purchase, so stock up on tuna packets or canned fish, so you always have a seafood source ready to go. For more guidance, the following shopping list offers suggestions for getting started on the pescatarian diet.

This sample shopping list is just an example of some things you might buy to follow the pescatarian diet. It is certainly not comprehensive, and many other foods are part of a nutrient-dense pescatarian diet.

- Dark leafy greens (spinach, kale, Swiss chard)
- Veggies (broccoli, cauliflower, Brussels sprouts, bell peppers, eggplant)
- Fresh and frozen fruits (grapefruit, oranges, berries, bananas, apples)
- Healthy fat sources (avocados, walnuts, almonds, chia seeds, olive oil)

- Whole grains (100% whole wheat bread, brown rice pasta, quinoa, barley)
- Plant-based protein and legumes (tofu, soybeans, black beans, lentils, chickpeas)
- Canned or packaged fish (tuna, sardines, anchovies, salmon, herring)
- Fresh or frozen fish (halibut, cod, salmon, snapper, sea bass)
- Dairy products (cheeses, yogurt, milk, cottage cheese)
- Eggs

PESCATARIAN DIET RECIPES COOKBOOK

Seared Salmon With Rosé and Herb Pan Sauce

Use rosé to make a simple pan sauce for seared wild salmon, and then enjoy a glass or two! The salmon cooks quickly, leaving lots of time for rosé all day.

contains Fin fish, Dairy

- PREP TIME 19 min COOK TIME 35 min TOTAL TIME 56 min

Ingredients

- 1½ cups rice, for serving
- 1 bunch trimmed asparagus, for serving
- 1 tbsp olive oil
- 2 6-oz portions skin-on wild salmon (center cut)
- Kosher salt and freshly ground pepper, to taste
- 1 lemon, halved
- 2 tbsp unsalted butter, divided
- 1 shallot, minced
- 1 tbsp fresh tarragon, chopped
- 1 tbsp fresh dill, chopped

- 1 tbsp fresh parsley, chopped

- 1 tbsp capers, rinsed

- ⅔ cup Bonterra rosé

Directions

1. Cook the rice: Cook rice to desired doneness according to package instructions. Keep warm until ready to serve.

2. Roast the asparagus: Preheat oven to 400 degrees F.

3. Arrange asparagus on a baking sheet and drizzle with olive oil. Season with salt and pepper to taste. Roast until lightly caramelized and crisp-tender, about 18 to 20 minutes. Keep warm until ready to serve.

4. Prepare the salmon: Meanwhile, season salmon on both sides with salt and pepper and let sit at room temperature for about 10 minutes.

5. In a coated cast-iron skillet or heavy-bottomed frying pan, add the olive oil and heat over medium high heat until shimmering. Add salmon (skin side up) and halved lemon and cook for about 4 minutes, or until salmon is golden brown and can

easily move around the pan. Remove lemon from
the pan and set aside on a plate. Flip salmon and
cook skin side down for another 3 minutes, then
add to the plate with the lemon and tent loosely
with foil.

6. Drain olive oil from the skillet and add 1 tbsp of
    butter. Once melted, add shallot and cook for about
    2 minutes or until they start to soften. Deglaze the
    pan with the rosé, scraping up brown bits from the
    bottom of the pan. Bring wine to a boil, then reduce
    heat and simmer until the liquid has reduced by
    half. Season with salt and pepper, then remove
    from heat.

7. Add the capers, herbs, and remaining 1 tbsp of
    butter and mount the sauce by slowly swirling the
    butter around in the pan.

8. Serve the salmon on top of prepared rice with
    roasted asparagus and a spoonful of the rosé pan
    sauce.

Nutrition Facts

Amount per serving

calories 527 total fat 31g saturated fat 10g protein 40g carbohydrates 9g fiber 0.9g sugar 5.2g added sugar 0g sodium 486mg

Grilled Octopus with Mediterranean Salad

! Here's a recipe for Grilled Octopus with Mediterranean Salad:

.Ingredients:.

For the Grilled Octopus:

- 1 whole octopus (about 2-3 pounds), cleaned and tentacles separated

- 1/4 cup olive oil

- 3 cloves garlic, minced

- Juice of 1 lemon

- Salt and black pepper to taste

- 1 teaspoon dried oregano

For the Mediterranean Salad:

- 1 cup cherry tomatoes, halved

- 1 cucumber, diced

- 1/2 red onion, thinly sliced

- 1/2 cup Kalamata olives, pitted and sliced

- 1/2 cup crumbled feta cheese

- 1/4 cup fresh parsley, chopped

- 2 tablespoons extra-virgin olive oil

- Juice of 1 lemon

- Salt and black pepper to taste

.Instructions:.

1. .Prepare the Octopus:.

   - In a large pot of boiling salted water, blanch the octopus for about 2-3 minutes to help tenderize it.

   - Remove the octopus from the boiling water and allow it to cool.

2. .Marinate the Octopus:.

   - In a bowl, whisk together the olive oil, minced garlic, lemon juice, dried oregano, salt, and black pepper.

- Add the cooled octopus to the marinade, ensuring it's well-coated. Marinate for at least 30 minutes or longer for better flavor.

3. .Grill the Octopus:.

   - Preheat your grill to medium-high heat.

   - Thread the octopus tentacles onto skewers or use a grill basket to prevent them from falling through the grates.

   - Grill the octopus for about 4-5 minutes per side until it develops grill marks and becomes tender. Be careful not to overcook, as it can become rubbery.

4. .Prepare the Mediterranean Salad:.

   - In a large bowl, combine the cherry tomatoes, cucumber, red onion, Kalamata olives, feta cheese, and fresh parsley.

   - In a small bowl, whisk together the extra-virgin olive oil, lemon juice, salt, and black pepper. Pour this dressing over the salad and toss to combine.

5. .Serve:.

   - Place the grilled octopus on a platter and serve it with the Mediterranean salad on the side.

This Grilled Octopus with Mediterranean Salad is a delightful and flavorful pescatarian dish that combines the smoky char of the octopus with the freshness of the salad. Enjoy!

Tofu and Vegetable Spring Rolls

! Here's a recipe for Tofu and Vegetable Spring Rolls with Peanut Dipping Sauce:

.Ingredients:.

For the Spring Rolls:

- 8 rice paper spring roll wrappers

- 8 small lettuce leaves (e.g., Bibb or Romaine)

- 1 cup thin rice noodles, cooked and cooled

- 1 cup firm tofu, thinly sliced into strips

- 1 cup cucumber, julienned

- 1 cup carrot, julienned

- 1/2 cup red bell pepper, thinly sliced

- 1/2 cup fresh cilantro leaves

- 1/4 cup fresh mint leaves

- 1/4 cup fresh basil leaves

For the Peanut Dipping Sauce:

- 1/2 cup creamy peanut butter

- 2 tablespoons soy sauce

- 2 tablespoons rice vinegar

- 1 tablespoon honey or maple syrup (for a vegan option)

- 1 clove garlic, minced

- 1/2 teaspoon grated fresh ginger

- 2-3 tablespoons warm water (to thin the sauce)

.Instructions:.

.Prepare the Peanut Dipping Sauce:.

1. In a bowl, whisk together peanut butter, soy sauce, rice vinegar, honey (or maple syrup), minced garlic, and grated ginger.
2. Gradually add warm water and whisk until you reach your desired dipping sauce consistency. Set the sauce aside.

.Assemble the Spring Rolls:.

3. Fill a shallow dish or pie plate with warm water. Dip one rice paper wrapper into the water for about 10-15 seconds until it becomes pliable.
4. Carefully transfer the soaked rice paper wrapper to a clean, damp kitchen towel.
5. Place a lettuce leaf on the lower third of the rice paper, leaving some space on each side.
6. Add a small amount of cooked rice noodles, tofu strips, cucumber, carrot, red bell pepper, cilantro, mint, and basil on top of the lettuce leaf.
7. Fold the sides of the rice paper over the filling, then gently roll up from the bottom, tucking in the sides as you go, to create a spring roll. Repeat with the remaining ingredients.
8. Place the finished spring rolls on a serving platter, seam side down.

.Serve:.

9. Serve the tofu and vegetable spring rolls with the peanut dipping sauce on the side. You can also garnish with additional herbs or crushed peanuts if desired.

These Tofu and Vegetable Spring Rolls with Peanut Dipping Sauce make for a refreshing and healthy pescatarian meal or snack. Enjoy!

Pesto Zucchini Noodles

! Here's a delicious recipe for Pesto Zucchini Noodles with Grilled Shrimp:

.Ingredients:.

For the Pesto:

- 2 cups fresh basil leaves, packed

- 1/2 cup grated Parmesan cheese

- 1/2 cup pine nuts

- 2 cloves garlic, minced

- 1/2 cup extra-virgin olive oil

- Salt and pepper to taste

- Juice of 1 lemon (optional, for added freshness)

For the Zucchini Noodles:

- 4 medium-sized zucchinis, spiralized into noodles

- 1 tablespoon olive oil

- Salt and pepper to taste

For the Grilled Shrimp:

- 1 pound large shrimp, peeled and deveined

- 2 tablespoons olive oil

- 2 cloves garlic, minced

- 1 teaspoon lemon zest

- Salt and pepper to taste

.Instructions:.

.Prepare the Pesto:.

1. In a food processor, combine the fresh basil, grated Parmesan cheese, pine nuts, and minced garlic.
2. Pulse the mixture until it's finely chopped.
3. With the food processor running, slowly drizzle in the extra-virgin olive oil until the pesto reaches your desired consistency.
4. Season the pesto with salt, pepper, and lemon juice (if using). Set it aside.

.Grill the Shrimp:.

5. In a bowl, combine the peeled and deveined shrimp with olive oil, minced garlic, lemon zest, salt, and pepper. Toss to coat the shrimp evenly.

6. Preheat your grill or grill pan to medium-high heat. Thread the shrimp onto skewers or use a grill basket.

7. Grill the shrimp for 2-3 minutes per side or until they turn pink and slightly charred. Remove them from the grill and set aside.

.Prepare the Zucchini Noodles:.

8. Heat 1 tablespoon of olive oil in a large skillet over medium heat.

9. Add the spiralized zucchini noodles and sauté for 2-3 minutes until they are just tender. Season with salt and pepper to taste.

.Assemble the Dish:.

10. Toss the sautéed zucchini noodles with the prepared pesto until they are well coated.

11. Arrange the pesto zucchini noodles on serving plates and top them with the grilled shrimp.

12. Garnish with extra grated Parmesan cheese and fresh basil leaves if desired.

Serve these Pesto Zucchini Noodles with Grilled Shrimp for a healthy and flavorful pescatarian meal. Enjoy!

Salmon and Avocado Salad

! Here's a recipe for a delicious Salmon and Avocado Salad with Sesame Dressing:

.Ingredients:.

For the Salad:

- 2 salmon fillets

- 1 tablespoon olive oil

- Salt and black pepper to taste

- 8 cups mixed salad greens (e.g., lettuce, spinach, arugula)

- 1 cucumber, thinly sliced

- 2 ripe avocados, sliced

- 1/4 cup red onion, thinly sliced

- 1/4 cup cherry tomatoes, halved

- 2 tablespoons sesame seeds, toasted

For the Sesame Dressing:

- 3 tablespoons sesame oil

- 2 tablespoons soy sauce

- 1 tablespoon rice vinegar

- 1 tablespoon honey or maple syrup (for a vegan option)

- 1 clove garlic, minced

- 1 teaspoon grated fresh ginger

- Salt and black pepper to taste

.Instructions:.

.Prepare the Salmon:.

1. Preheat your oven to 375°F (190°C).
2. Place the salmon fillets on a baking sheet lined with parchment paper.
3. Drizzle olive oil over the salmon and season with salt and black pepper.
4. Bake the salmon in the preheated oven for 12-15 minutes or until it flakes easily with a fork. Remove from the oven and let it cool slightly.
5. Once cooled, break the salmon into large flakes with a fork.

.Make the Sesame Dressing:.

6. In a small bowl, whisk together the sesame oil, soy
    sauce, rice vinegar, honey (or maple syrup), minced
    garlic, grated ginger, salt, and black pepper. Adjust
    the seasoning to your taste.

.Assemble the Salad:.

7. In a large salad bowl, combine the mixed greens,
    sliced cucumber, avocado slices, red onion, and
    cherry tomatoes.
8. Drizzle the sesame dressing over the salad and toss
    gently to coat the ingredients.
9. Top the salad with the flaked salmon and toasted
    sesame seeds.

.Serve:.

10. Divide the Salmon and Avocado Salad among
    individual plates.
11. Serve immediately, garnished with extra sesame
    seeds if desired.

This Salmon and Avocado Salad with Sesame Dressing is
a delightful combination of flavors and textures, making
it a perfect choice for a healthy pescatarian meal. Enjoy!

Teriyaki Tempeh and Vegetable Skewers

! Here's a recipe for Teriyaki Tempeh and Vegetable Skewers:

.Ingredients:.

For the Teriyaki Marinade:

- 1/2 cup soy sauce

- 1/4 cup water

- 2 tablespoons rice vinegar

- 2 tablespoons honey or maple syrup (for a vegan option)

- 1 clove garlic, minced

- 1 teaspoon grated fresh ginger

- 1 tablespoon cornstarch (to thicken)

- 1 tablespoon water (for cornstarch mixture)

For the Skewers:

- 1 block (8 ounces) tempeh, cut into cubes

- Assorted vegetables, cut into bite-sized pieces (e.g., bell peppers, zucchini, red onion, mushrooms, cherry tomatoes)

- Wooden skewers, soaked in water for 30 minutes (to prevent burning)

- 2 tablespoons vegetable oil (for grilling)

- Sesame seeds and chopped green onions for garnish (optional)

.Instructions:.

.Prepare the Teriyaki Marinade:.

1. In a saucepan, combine the soy sauce, water, rice vinegar, honey (or maple syrup), minced garlic, and grated ginger. Heat over medium heat and bring to a simmer.
2. In a small bowl, mix the cornstarch with 1 tablespoon of water to create a cornstarch mixture.
3. Slowly whisk the cornstarch mixture into the simmering sauce. Continue to simmer for 1-2 minutes, or until the sauce thickens. Remove it from heat and set aside.

.Marinate the Tempeh and Vegetables:.

4. In a shallow dish or large resealable bag, pour half of the teriyaki marinade over the cubed tempeh.

Allow it to marinate for at least 30 minutes, or longer for more flavor.

5. Thread the marinated tempeh and assorted vegetables onto the soaked wooden skewers, alternating between them.

    1. .Grill the Skewers:.

6. Preheat your grill to medium-high heat.

7. Brush the skewers with vegetable oil to prevent sticking.

8. Grill the skewers for about 3-4 minutes per side, basting them with the reserved teriyaki marinade as they cook. Continue grilling until the tempeh and vegetables are nicely charred and cooked to your liking.

.Serve:.

9. Remove the skewers from the grill and place them on a serving platter.

10. Garnish with sesame seeds and chopped green onions if desired.

These Teriyaki Tempeh and Vegetable Skewers are a flavorful and satisfying pescatarian option that's perfect for a barbecue or outdoor meal. Enjoy!

Smoked Haddock and Potato Chowder

! Here's a recipe for Smoked Haddock and Potato Chowder:

.Ingredients:.

- 1 pound (450g) smoked haddock fillets

- 2 tablespoons butter

- 1 onion, diced

- 2 cloves garlic, minced

- 2 celery stalks, diced

- 2 carrots, diced

- 2 cups (about 450g) potatoes, peeled and diced into small cubes

- 4 cups (946ml) chicken or vegetable broth

- 1 bay leaf

- 1 teaspoon dried thyme

- 1 cup (240ml) heavy cream

- Salt and black pepper to taste

- Fresh parsley, chopped (for garnish)

.Prepare the Smoked Haddock:.

1. Place the smoked haddock fillets in a shallow dish and cover them with milk. Let them soak for about 20-30 minutes. This helps to reduce the smoky saltiness of the fish.
2. After soaking, remove the haddock from the milk, pat them dry with paper towels, and cut them into small chunks. Set aside.

.Make the Chowder:.

3. In a large pot, melt the butter over medium heat.
4. Add the diced onion, garlic, celery, and carrots. Sauté for about 5-7 minutes, or until the vegetables become tender.
5. Add the diced potatoes, chicken or vegetable broth, bay leaf, and dried thyme to the pot. Bring the mixture to a boil, then reduce the heat to a simmer. Cover and cook for about 10-15 minutes, or until the potatoes are tender.
6. Once the potatoes are tender, remove the bay leaf from the pot.

7. Use an immersion blender to partially blend the chowder, leaving some chunks for texture. Alternatively, remove about half of the chowder and blend it in a blender, then return it to the pot.

8. Stir in the heavy cream and the chunks of smoked haddock.

9. Simmer the chowder for an additional 5-7 minutes, or until the haddock is cooked through and flakes easily.

10. Season the chowder with salt and black pepper to taste. Adjust the seasoning as needed.

.Serve:.

11. Ladle the smoked haddock and potato chowder into bowls.

12. Garnish with fresh chopped parsley.

This Smoked Haddock and Potato Chowder is a comforting and flavorful pescatarian dish, perfect for a cozy meal on a chilly day. Enjoy!

Spaghetti Aglio e Olio

! Here's a recipe for Spaghetti Aglio e Olio with Anchovies:

.Ingredients:.

- 12 ounces (340g) spaghetti

- 1/4 cup extra-virgin olive oil

- 4-6 cloves garlic, thinly sliced

- 4-6 anchovy fillets (adjust to taste)

- 1/4 to 1/2 teaspoon red pepper flakes (adjust to taste)

- Salt and black pepper to taste

- 1/4 cup fresh parsley, chopped

- Grated Parmesan cheese for garnish (optional)

.Instructions:.

1. Cook the Spaghetti:

   - Cook the spaghetti in a large pot of salted boiling water according to the package instructions until al dente. Drain and set aside, reserving about 1/2 cup of pasta cooking water.

2. Prepare the Anchovy and Garlic Mixture:

- In a large skillet, heat the extra-virgin olive oil over medium heat.

- Add the thinly sliced garlic and cook for about 1-2 minutes until it becomes fragrant and just starts to turn golden.

3. Add the Anchovies and Red Pepper Flakes:

- Add the anchovy fillets to the skillet. Use a spatula or fork to break them apart and let them dissolve into the oil.

- Sprinkle the red pepper flakes into the skillet, adjusting the amount to your preferred level of spiciness. Stir and cook for another minute.

4. Combine Spaghetti and Sauce:

- Add the cooked and drained spaghetti to the skillet with the anchovy and garlic mixture.

- Toss the pasta in the sauce until it's well coated. If it seems a bit dry, add some of the reserved pasta cooking water to reach your desired consistency.

5. Season and Garnish:

- Season the spaghetti with salt and black pepper to taste. Remember that anchovies are naturally salty, so go easy on the salt until you've tasted the dish.

- Stir in the chopped fresh parsley and toss everything together.

6. Serve:

  - Divide the Spaghetti Aglio e Olio with Anchovies among serving plates.

  - If desired, garnish with grated Parmesan cheese.

This Spaghetti Aglio e Olio with Anchovies is a simple yet flavorful pescatarian pasta dish with a delightful combination of garlic, anchovies, and a touch of heat from the red pepper flakes. Enjoy!

Stuffed Acorn Squash with Quinoa

! Here's a recipe for Stuffed Acorn Squash with Quinoa and Shrimp:

.Ingredients:.

For the Acorn Squash:

- 2 acorn squash, halved and seeds removed

- 2 tablespoons olive oil

- Salt and black pepper to taste

For the Filling:

- 1 cup quinoa, rinsed and drained

- 2 cups vegetable broth or water

- 1 pound large shrimp, peeled and deveined

- 2 tablespoons olive oil

- 1 onion, finely chopped

- 2 cloves garlic, minced

- 1 red bell pepper, diced

- 1 zucchini, diced

- 1/2 cup frozen peas

- 1 teaspoon dried thyme

- Salt and black pepper to taste

- 1/4 cup chopped fresh parsley

- Juice of 1 lemon

.Instructions:.

.Prepare the Acorn Squash:.

1. Preheat your oven to 400°F (200°C).
2. Brush the cut sides of the acorn squash halves with olive oil and season with salt and black pepper.

3. Place the squash halves, cut side down, on a baking sheet lined with parchment paper.

4. Bake in the preheated oven for about 30-40 minutes or until the squash is tender when pierced with a fork. Remove from the oven and set aside.

.Prepare the Quinoa:.

5. In a saucepan, combine the rinsed quinoa and vegetable broth (or water). Bring to a boil, then reduce the heat to low, cover, and simmer for about 15-20 minutes, or until the quinoa is cooked and the liquid is absorbed. Remove from heat and fluff with a fork.

.Prepare the Shrimp and Vegetable Filling:.

6. Heat 2 tablespoons of olive oil in a large skillet over medium-high heat.

7. Add the chopped onion and cook for 2-3 minutes until it becomes translucent.

8. Stir in the minced garlic and cook for another 30 seconds until fragrant.

9. Add the diced red bell pepper, zucchini, and frozen peas to the skillet. Sauté for about 5 minutes or until the vegetables are tender.

10. Add the shrimp and dried thyme to the skillet. Cook for 2-3 minutes on each side or until the shrimp turn pink and opaque.

11. Stir the cooked quinoa into the skillet with the shrimp and vegetables. Mix well to combine.

12. Season the filling with salt, black pepper, chopped fresh parsley, and lemon juice. Adjust the seasoning to your taste.

.Assemble and Serve:.

13. Fill each roasted acorn squash half with the quinoa and shrimp mixture.

14. Garnish with extra chopped parsley if desired.

These Stuffed Acorn Squash with Quinoa and Shrimp make for a hearty and flavorful pescatarian dish that's perfect for a satisfying meal. Enjoy!

Shrimp and Broccoli Alfredo

! Here's a recipe for Shrimp and Broccoli Alfredo:

.Ingredients:.

- 8 ounces (about 2 cups) fettuccine pasta

- 1 pound large shrimp, peeled and deveined

- 2 cups broccoli florets

- 2 tablespoons butter

- 2 cloves garlic, minced

- 1 cup heavy cream

- 1 cup grated Parmesan cheese

- Salt and black pepper to taste

- Fresh parsley, chopped (for garnish, optional)

.Instructions:.

1. .Cook the Fettuccine:.

   - Cook the fettuccine pasta in a large pot of salted boiling water according to the package instructions until al dente. Drain and set aside.

2. .Prepare the Shrimp and Broccoli:.

   - In a large skillet, melt 1 tablespoon of butter over medium heat.

   - Add the minced garlic and sauté for about 30 seconds until fragrant.

   - Add the shrimp to the skillet and cook for 2-3 minutes on each side or until they turn pink and opaque. Remove the cooked shrimp from the skillet and set them aside.

   - In the same skillet, add the remaining 1 tablespoon of butter and the broccoli florets. Sauté the broccoli for about 3-4 minutes until they become tender.

3. .Make the Alfredo Sauce:.

   - Reduce the heat to low, and pour in the heavy cream. Stir well to combine.

   - Gradually add the grated Parmesan cheese to the cream, stirring continuously until the cheese is fully melted and the sauce thickens.

4. .Combine Everything:.

   - Return the cooked shrimp to the skillet with the broccoli and Alfredo sauce.

   - Add the cooked fettuccine pasta to the skillet as well.

5. .Season and Serve:.

   - Gently toss all the ingredients in the skillet to coat them with the creamy Alfredo sauce.

   - Season with salt and black pepper to taste.

   - If desired, garnish with chopped fresh parsley.

6. .Serve immediately.while the Shrimp and Broccoli Alfredo is hot.

This Shrimp and Broccoli Alfredo is a creamy and indulgent pescatarian dish that's perfect for a comforting meal. Enjoy!

Citrus Glazed Grilled Salmon

! Here's a recipe for Citrus Glazed Grilled Salmon:

.Ingredients:.

For the Citrus Glaze:

- 1/4 cup orange juice

- 2 tablespoons lemon juice

- 2 tablespoons lime juice

- 1/4 cup honey

- 2 cloves garlic, minced

- 1 teaspoon grated orange zest

- 1 teaspoon grated lemon zest

- Salt and black pepper to taste

For the Grilled Salmon:

- 4 salmon fillets (6-8 ounces each)

- 2 tablespoons olive oil

- Salt and black pepper to taste

- Fresh parsley or cilantro, chopped (for garnish, optional)

.Instructions:.

.Prepare the Citrus Glaze:.

1. In a small saucepan, combine the orange juice, lemon juice, lime juice, honey, minced garlic, grated orange zest, and grated lemon zest.
2. Place the saucepan over medium heat and bring the mixture to a simmer.
3. Reduce the heat to low and simmer for about 5-7 minutes, stirring occasionally, until the glaze thickens and becomes glossy.
4. Season the glaze with salt and black pepper to taste. Remove it from the heat and set it aside.

.Prepare and Grill the Salmon:.

5. Preheat your grill to medium-high heat and oil the grates to prevent sticking.
6. Brush the salmon fillets with olive oil and season them with salt and black pepper.

7. Place the salmon fillets on the preheated grill, skin-side down.

8. Grill the salmon for about 4-5 minutes on the first side. Use a spatula to carefully flip the fillets over.

9. Brush the grilled side of the salmon with the prepared citrus glaze.

10. Continue grilling for another 4-5 minutes or until the salmon is cooked through and easily flakes with a fork. Brush the salmon with more citrus glaze during grilling.

.Serve:.

11. Remove the grilled salmon from the grill and place it on a serving platter.

12. Drizzle any remaining citrus glaze over the salmon fillets.

13. If desired, garnish with chopped fresh parsley or cilantro.

This Citrus Glazed Grilled Salmon is a flavorful and vibrant pescatarian dish with a perfect balance of sweet and tangy flavors. Enjoy!

Tofu and Vegetable Thai Green Curry

! Here's a recipe for Tofu and Vegetable Thai Green Curry:

.Ingredients:.

For the Green Curry Paste:

- 2-3 green Thai chilies (adjust to your spice preference)

- 2 stalks lemongrass, chopped (use only the bottom white part)

- 3 cloves garlic, minced

- 1 small onion, chopped

- 1 thumb-sized piece of ginger, peeled and chopped

- 2 tablespoons fresh cilantro leaves and stems

- 1 tablespoon fresh basil leaves

- 1 teaspoon ground cumin

- 1 teaspoon ground coriander

- 1/2 teaspoon ground white pepper

- Zest and juice of 1 lime

- 2-3 tablespoons water (as needed)

For the Curry:

- 14 ounces (400g) extra-firm tofu, cubed

- 2 tablespoons vegetable oil

- 1 can (14 ounces) coconut milk

- 1 cup broccoli florets

- 1 cup sliced bell peppers (red, green, or yellow)

- 1 cup sliced carrots

- 1 cup sliced zucchini

- 1 cup sliced mushrooms

- 2 tablespoons soy sauce

- 1 tablespoon brown sugar (or palm sugar)

- Salt, to taste

- Fresh basil leaves and lime wedges for garnish

- Cooked jasmine rice or rice noodles (for serving)

.Instructions:.

.Prepare the Green Curry Paste:.

1. In a food processor or blender, combine all the
    ingredients for the green curry paste. Blend until

you have a smooth paste, adding water as needed
to achieve the right consistency. Set the paste aside.

.Prepare the Tofu:.

2. In a large skillet or wok, heat the vegetable oil over
    medium-high heat.

3. Add the tofu cubes and stir-fry for about 3-4
    minutes until they become lightly golden. Remove
    the tofu from the skillet and set it aside.

.Make the Curry:.

4. In the same skillet, add a little more oil if needed
    and then add 3-4 tablespoons of the green curry
    paste (adjust to your desired level of spiciness).

5. Sauté the green curry paste for 1-2 minutes until it
    becomes fragrant.

6. Pour in the coconut milk and stir to combine with
    the curry paste.

7. Add the broccoli, bell peppers, carrots, zucchini, and
    mushrooms to the skillet. Stir to coat the vegetables
    with the curry sauce.

8. Cover the skillet and let the vegetables simmer in
    the sauce for about 10-12 minutes, or until they
    become tender.

9. Stir in the soy sauce and brown sugar. Adjust the seasoning with salt if needed.

10. Add the stir-fried tofu back into the skillet and gently combine it with the vegetables and sauce.

.Serve:.

11. Serve the Tofu and Vegetable Thai Green Curry hot, garnished with fresh basil leaves and lime wedges.

12. Serve with cooked jasmine rice or rice noodles.

Enjoy your homemade Tofu and Vegetable Thai Green Curry, a delicious and aromatic pescatarian dish!

Baked Red Snapper with Chimichurri Sauce

! Here's a recipe for Baked Red Snapper with Chimichurri Sauce:

.Ingredients:.

For the Baked Red Snapper:

- 4 red snapper fillets (about 6-8 ounces each)

- 2 tablespoons olive oil

- Salt and black pepper to taste

- 1 lemon, thinly sliced

- Fresh parsley or cilantro leaves for garnish

For the Chimichurri Sauce:

- 1 cup fresh parsley leaves, chopped

- 1/4 cup fresh cilantro leaves, chopped

- 3 cloves garlic, minced

- 1 shallot, finely chopped

- 1 red chili pepper, seeded and finely chopped (adjust to taste)

- 1 teaspoon dried oregano

- 1/2 cup extra-virgin olive oil

- 2 tablespoons red wine vinegar

- Juice of 1 lemon

- Salt and black pepper to taste

.Instructions:.

.Prepare the Chimichurri Sauce:.

1. In a bowl, combine the chopped fresh parsley, cilantro, minced garlic, chopped shallot, chopped red chili pepper, and dried oregano.

2. Stir in the extra-virgin olive oil, red wine vinegar, and lemon juice.

3. Season the chimichurri sauce with salt and black pepper to taste. Adjust the seasoning as needed.

4. Set the chimichurri sauce aside to allow the flavors to meld while you prepare the red snapper.

.Bake the Red Snapper:.

5. Preheat your oven to 400°F (200°C).

6. Place the red snapper fillets on a baking sheet lined with parchment paper or in a baking dish.

7. Brush each fillet with olive oil and season with salt and black pepper.

8. Arrange lemon slices on top of the snapper fillets.

9. Bake the red snapper in the preheated oven for about 15-20 minutes, or until the fish is opaque and flakes easily with a fork.

.Serve:.

10. Remove the baked red snapper from the oven and transfer it to serving plates.

11. Spoon the prepared chimichurri sauce generously over each fillet.

12. Garnish with fresh parsley or cilantro leaves.

Serve your Baked Red Snapper with Chimichurri Sauce hot, with your choice of side dishes like rice, quinoa, or steamed vegetables. Enjoy this flavorful and colorful pescatarian dish!

Vegan Lentil and Chickpea Curry

! Here's a recipe for Vegan Lentil and Chickpea Curry:

.Ingredients:.

- 1 cup dried green or brown lentils, rinsed and drained

- 1 can (15 ounces) chickpeas, drained and rinsed

- 2 tablespoons olive oil

- 1 large onion, chopped

- 3 cloves garlic, minced

- 1-inch piece of fresh ginger, grated

- 2 tablespoons curry powder (adjust to taste)

- 1 teaspoon ground turmeric

- 1 teaspoon ground cumin

- 1 teaspoon ground coriander

- 1 can (14 ounces) diced tomatoes

- 1 can (14 ounces) coconut milk

- 2 cups vegetable broth

- 2 cups chopped spinach or kale

- Salt and black pepper to taste

- Fresh cilantro leaves for garnish (optional)

- Cooked rice or naan bread (for serving)

.Instructions:.

.Cook the Lentils and Chickpeas:.

1. In a medium-sized pot, combine the rinsed lentils with enough water to cover them by about 2 inches. Bring to a boil, then reduce the heat to a simmer and cook for about 15-20 minutes or until the lentils are tender but not mushy. Drain any excess water.

2. In a separate pot, add the chickpeas and enough water to cover them. Bring to a boil, then reduce the heat and simmer for about 10 minutes. Drain and set aside.

.Prepare the Curry:.

3. In a large skillet or pan, heat the olive oil over medium heat.

4. Add the chopped onion and sauté for about 5 minutes until it becomes translucent.

5. Stir in the minced garlic and grated ginger and cook for another minute until fragrant.

6. Add the curry powder, ground turmeric, ground cumin, and ground coriander to the skillet. Cook for 1-2 minutes, stirring continuously until the spices are toasted and fragrant.

7. Pour in the diced tomatoes (with their juices) and coconut milk. Stir to combine.

8. Add the cooked lentils, chickpeas, and vegetable broth to the skillet. Mix well.

9. Bring the mixture to a simmer and let it cook for about 15-20 minutes, allowing the flavors to meld and the sauce to thicken.

10. Stir in the chopped spinach or kale and cook for an additional 3-5 minutes until the greens are wilted.

11. Season the vegan lentil and chickpea curry with salt and black pepper to taste. Adjust the seasoning as needed.

.Serve:.

12. Serve the Vegan Lentil and Chickpea Curry hot, garnished with fresh cilantro leaves if desired.
13. Serve with cooked rice or naan bread for a complete and satisfying meal.

Enjoy your homemade Vegan Lentil and Chickpea Curry, a flavorful and nutritious plant-based dish!

Creamy Mushroom and Spinach Risotto

! Here's a recipe for Creamy Mushroom and Spinach Risotto with Shrimp:

.Ingredients:.

For the Risotto:

- 1 1/2 cups Arborio rice

- 8 cups vegetable or chicken broth (kept hot)

- 1 cup dry white wine (optional)

- 2 tablespoons olive oil

- 1 small onion, finely chopped

- 2 cloves garlic, minced

- 8 ounces (about 2 cups) mushrooms, sliced (button, cremini, or wild mushrooms)

- 1 cup baby spinach leaves

- 1/2 cup grated Parmesan cheese

- Salt and black pepper to taste

- Fresh parsley, chopped (for garnish, optional)

For the Shrimp:

- 1 pound large shrimp, peeled and deveined

- 2 tablespoons olive oil

- 2 cloves garlic, minced

- Salt and black pepper to taste

- Lemon wedges (for garnish)

.Instructions:.

.Prepare the Shrimp:.

1. In a large skillet, heat 2 tablespoons of olive oil over medium-high heat.
2. Add the minced garlic and sauté for about 30 seconds until fragrant.
3. Add the peeled and deveined shrimp to the skillet.

4. Season the shrimp with salt and black pepper to taste.

5. Cook the shrimp for about 2-3 minutes per side, or until they turn pink and opaque. Remove them from the skillet and set aside.

.Make the Risotto:.

6. In a large, deep skillet or a wide saucepan, heat 2 tablespoons of olive oil over medium heat.

7. Add the finely chopped onion and sauté for about 3-4 minutes until it becomes translucent.

8. Stir in the minced garlic and cook for another 30 seconds until fragrant.

9. Add the sliced mushrooms to the skillet and cook for about 5-7 minutes until they release their moisture and start to brown.

10. Add the Arborio rice to the skillet and stir to coat the rice with the mushroom mixture.

11. If using, pour in the white wine and stir until it's mostly absorbed by the rice.

12. Begin adding the hot vegetable or chicken broth, one ladle at a time, stirring constantly. Allow each ladle of broth to be absorbed by the rice before

adding more. Continue this process until the rice is creamy and cooked to your desired level of doneness (usually about 18-20 minutes).

13. Stir in the grated Parmesan cheese until it's fully melted into the risotto.

14. Gently fold in the baby spinach leaves and cook until they wilt and become incorporated into the risotto.

15. Season the risotto with salt and black pepper to taste. Adjust the seasoning as needed.

.Serve:.

16. Divide the Creamy Mushroom and Spinach Risotto among serving plates.

17. Top each serving with the cooked shrimp.

18. Garnish with fresh chopped parsley and serve with lemon wedges on the side.

Enjoy your homemade Creamy Mushroom and Spinach Risotto with Shrimp, a delightful and satisfying pescatarian dish!

Grilled Trout with Lemon

! Here's a recipe for Grilled Trout with Lemon and Herbs:

.Ingredients:

For the Grilled Trout:

- 4 whole trout, cleaned and gutted

- 2 tablespoons olive oil

- Salt and black pepper to taste

- 2 lemons, thinly sliced

- Fresh herbs (such as thyme, rosemary, or parsley), for garnish

- Lemon wedges, for serving

For the Lemon-Herb Marinade:

- 1/4 cup fresh lemon juice

- Zest of 1 lemon

- 3 cloves garlic, minced

- 2 tablespoons fresh parsley, chopped

- 2 tablespoons fresh thyme leaves (or other herbs of your choice)

- 2 tablespoons olive oil

- Salt and black pepper to taste

.Instructions:.

.Prepare the Lemon-Herb Marinade:.

1. In a bowl, combine the fresh lemon juice, lemon zest, minced garlic, chopped parsley, thyme leaves (or other herbs of your choice), and olive oil.
2. Season the marinade with salt and black pepper to taste. Mix well.

.Marinate and Grill the Trout:.

3. Place the cleaned and gutted trout in a shallow dish or a resealable plastic bag.
4. Pour the lemon-herb marinade over the trout, making sure each fish is well coated. You can also stuff some of the herbs and lemon slices into the cavities of the fish for extra flavor.
5. Cover the dish or seal the bag and refrigerate for at least 30 minutes, allowing the trout to marinate.
6. Preheat your grill to medium-high heat and oil the grates to prevent sticking.

7. Remove the trout from the marinade and let any excess marinade drip off.

8. Season the trout with salt and black pepper, and brush both sides with olive oil.

9. Place the trout on the preheated grill, skin-side down.

10. Grill the trout for about 4-5 minutes per side, or until the flesh flakes easily with a fork and has a nice grill mark.

.Serve:.

11. Transfer the grilled trout to a serving platter.

12. Garnish with fresh herbs and lemon wedges.

13. Serve your Grilled Trout with Lemon and Herbs hot, with your choice of side dishes like grilled vegetables or a salad.

Enjoy this flavorful and fresh grilled trout with the zesty goodness of lemon and herbs!

Vegetarian Kimchi Fried Rice

! Here's a recipe for Vegetarian Kimchi Fried Rice with Tofu:

.Ingredients:.

- 2 cups cooked and cooled rice (preferably day-old)

- 8 ounces (about 1/2 block) firm tofu, cubed

- 1 cup kimchi, chopped

- 2 tablespoons kimchi juice (from the jar)

- 2 tablespoons vegetable oil

- 1 small onion, finely chopped

- 2 cloves garlic, minced

- 1 carrot, diced

- 1 cup frozen peas

- 2 tablespoons soy sauce

- 1 tablespoon sesame oil

- 1 green onion, chopped (for garnish)

- Toasted sesame seeds (for garnish, optional)

.Prepare the Tofu:.

1.   Place the cubed tofu between paper towels and press gently to remove excess moisture. You can also use a tofu press if you have one.

2.   Heat 1 tablespoon of vegetable oil in a large skillet or wok over medium-high heat.

3.   Add the cubed tofu to the skillet and cook for about 4-5 minutes, turning occasionally, until it becomes golden and crispy on all sides. Remove the tofu from the skillet and set it aside.

.Make the Kimchi Fried Rice:.

4.   In the same skillet, add the remaining 1 tablespoon of vegetable oil.

5.   Add the chopped onion and garlic to the skillet and sauté for about 2-3 minutes until the onion becomes translucent.

6.   Stir in the diced carrot and frozen peas. Cook for another 3-4 minutes until the vegetables begin to soften.

7. Add the chopped kimchi and kimchi juice to the skillet. Stir-fry for 2-3 minutes to incorporate the kimchi flavors with the vegetables.

8. Add the cooked and cooled rice to the skillet. Break up any clumps and stir-fry for about 5 minutes until the rice is heated through and starts to turn slightly crispy.

9. Pour in the soy sauce and sesame oil, and stir to evenly distribute the seasonings.

10. Gently fold in the cooked tofu cubes and cook for an additional 2-3 minutes to warm the tofu.

.Serve:.

11. Remove the Vegetarian Kimchi Fried Rice with Tofu from the heat.

12. Garnish with chopped green onions and toasted sesame seeds if desired.

Serve your flavorful Vegetarian Kimchi Fried Rice with Tofu hot, and enjoy the combination of spicy kimchi, crispy tofu, and aromatic seasonings!

Scallops in Garlic Butter Sauce

! Here's a recipe for Scallops in Garlic Butter Sauce:

.Ingredients:.

- 1 pound fresh scallops

- 2 tablespoons unsalted butter

- 2 tablespoons olive oil

- 4 cloves garlic, minced

- 1/4 cup dry white wine (optional)

- Juice of 1 lemon

- Salt and black pepper to taste

- Fresh parsley, chopped, for garnish (optional)

- Lemon wedges, for serving

.Instructions:.

.Prepare the Scallops:.

1. Pat the scallops dry with paper towels to remove excess moisture.

2. Season both sides of the scallops with a pinch of salt and black pepper.

.Cook the Scallops:.

3. In a large skillet, heat the olive oil and butter over medium-high heat.

4. Add the minced garlic to the skillet and sauté for about 30 seconds until fragrant, being careful not to let it brown.

5. Carefully add the seasoned scallops to the skillet in a single layer, making sure not to overcrowd them. You may need to cook them in batches if your skillet is not large enough.

6. Cook the scallops for about 2-3 minutes on each side, or until they turn golden brown and develop a nice sear. Avoid overcooking, as scallops can become tough if cooked too long. They should be opaque and slightly translucent in the center when done.

.Create the Garlic Butter Sauce:.

7. If using, pour the white wine into the skillet and stir to deglaze the pan, scraping up any browned bits from the bottom.

8. Add the lemon juice to the skillet and stir it into the butter sauce.

9. Taste the sauce and adjust the seasoning with salt
    and black pepper if needed.

.Serve:.

10. Remove the scallops from the skillet and place them
    on serving plates.

11. Pour the garlic butter sauce over the scallops.

12. Garnish with chopped fresh parsley if desired.

13. Serve your Scallops in Garlic Butter Sauce hot, with
    lemon wedges on the side.

Enjoy your delicious Scallops in Garlic Butter Sauce, a
simple yet elegant seafood dish!

Tuna and White Bean Salad

! Here's a recipe for Tuna and White Bean Salad:

.Ingredients:.

For the Salad:

- 2 cans (15 ounces each) white beans (cannellini or
Great Northern), drained and rinsed

- 2 cans (5 ounces each) tuna in olive oil, drained and
flaked

- 1/2 red onion, finely chopped

- 1/2 cup cherry tomatoes, halved

- 1/4 cup fresh parsley, chopped

- 1/4 cup black olives, pitted and sliced (optional)

- Salt and black pepper to taste

For the Dressing:

- 3 tablespoons extra-virgin olive oil

- 2 tablespoons red wine vinegar

- 1 clove garlic, minced

- 1 teaspoon Dijon mustard

- Salt and black pepper to taste

.Instructions:.

.Prepare the Salad:.

1. In a large bowl, combine the drained and rinsed white beans, flaked tuna, finely chopped red onion, halved cherry tomatoes, chopped fresh parsley, and sliced black olives (if using).

2. Gently toss the salad ingredients to combine.

.Make the Dressing:.

3. In a separate bowl, whisk together the extra-virgin olive oil, red wine vinegar, minced garlic, Dijon mustard, salt, and black pepper to taste. Whisk until well combined.

.Combine and Serve:.

4. Pour the dressing over the tuna and white bean salad.
5. Gently toss the salad to coat the ingredients with the dressing.
6. Taste and adjust the seasoning with more salt and black pepper if needed.
7. Allow the salad to chill in the refrigerator for about 15-30 minutes before serving to let the flavors meld.
8. Serve your Tuna and White Bean Salad chilled as a refreshing and nutritious dish.

This Tuna and White Bean Salad is a satisfying and protein-packed option, perfect for a light meal or as a side dish. Enjoy!

Spicy Sriracha Tofu Stir-Fry

! Here's a recipe for Spicy Sriracha Tofu Stir-Fry:

.Ingredients:.

For the Sriracha Tofu:

- 14 ounces (about 1 block) extra-firm tofu, cubed

- 2 tablespoons Sriracha sauce

- 2 tablespoons soy sauce

- 2 cloves garlic, minced

- 1 tablespoon sesame oil

- 1 tablespoon olive oil

- Salt and black pepper to taste

For the Stir-Fry:

- 2 tablespoons vegetable oil

- 1 small onion, thinly sliced

- 1 bell pepper, thinly sliced (any color)

- 1 cup broccoli florets

- 1 carrot, thinly sliced

- 1 cup snap peas, trimmed

- 1/2 cup baby corn, cut into bite-sized pieces

- 2-3 green onions, chopped (for garnish)

- Cooked rice or noodles (for serving)

.Instructions:.

.Prepare the Sriracha Tofu:.

1. In a bowl, combine the Sriracha sauce, soy sauce, minced garlic, sesame oil, olive oil, salt, and black pepper.
2. Add the cubed tofu to the bowl and gently toss to coat the tofu with the Sriracha mixture. Allow it to marinate for at least 15 minutes.

.Stir-Fry the Vegetables:.

3. Heat 2 tablespoons of vegetable oil in a large skillet or wok over medium-high heat.
4. Add the thinly sliced onion and stir-fry for about 2-3 minutes until it becomes translucent.
5. Add the thinly sliced bell pepper, broccoli florets, sliced carrot, snap peas, and baby corn to the skillet. Stir-fry for 5-7 minutes, or until the vegetables are tender-crisp.

.Cook the Sriracha Tofu:.

6. Push the cooked vegetables to one side of the skillet.
7. In the empty side of the skillet, add the marinated Sriracha tofu and any remaining marinade.
8. Cook the tofu for about 3-4 minutes on each side, or until it becomes golden and slightly crispy.

.Combine and Serve:.

9. Gently combine the cooked tofu with the stir-fried vegetables in the skillet.
10. Taste and adjust the seasoning, adding more Sriracha sauce or soy sauce if desired.
11. Serve your Spicy Sriracha Tofu Stir-Fry hot, garnished with chopped green onions, and with cooked rice or noodles on the side.

Enjoy your Spicy Sriracha Tofu Stir-Fry, a flavorful and spicy vegetarian dish!

Baked Cod with Mediterranean Tomato Sauce

! Here's a recipe for Baked Cod with Mediterranean Tomato Sauce:

.Ingredients:.

For the Cod:

- 4 cod fillets (about 6 ounces each)

- 2 tablespoons olive oil

- Salt and black pepper to taste

- 1 lemon, thinly sliced

- Fresh parsley, chopped, for garnish

For the Mediterranean Tomato Sauce:

- 1 tablespoon olive oil

- 1 small onion, finely chopped

- 2 cloves garlic, minced

- 1 can (14 ounces) diced tomatoes (preferably fire-roasted)

- 1/4 cup Kalamata olives, pitted and sliced

- 1/4 cup artichoke hearts, chopped

- 1/4 cup sun-dried tomatoes, chopped

- 1 teaspoon dried oregano

- 1/2 teaspoon dried basil

- Salt and black pepper to taste

- Crushed red pepper flakes (optional, for heat)

- Fresh basil leaves, for garnish (optional)

.Instructions:.

.Prepare the Mediterranean Tomato Sauce:.

1. In a saucepan, heat 1 tablespoon of olive oil over medium heat.
2. Add the finely chopped onion and sauté for about 3-4 minutes until it becomes translucent.
3. Stir in the minced garlic and cook for another 30 seconds until fragrant.
4. Add the diced tomatoes (with their juices), Kalamata olives, chopped artichoke hearts, chopped sun-dried tomatoes, dried oregano, dried basil, salt, and black pepper to the saucepan. If you like a bit of heat, add some crushed red pepper flakes.

5. Simmer the sauce for about 10-15 minutes, stirring occasionally, until it thickens and the flavors meld. Adjust the seasoning if needed.

.Prepare the Baked Cod:.

6. Preheat your oven to 375°F (190°C).
7. Place the cod fillets on a baking sheet lined with parchment paper or in a baking dish.
8. Brush each fillet with 2 tablespoons of olive oil and season with salt and black pepper.
9. Arrange lemon slices on top of the cod fillets.

.Bake:.

10. Bake the cod in the preheated oven for about 12-15 minutes, or until the fish flakes easily with a fork and is opaque in the center.

.Serve:.

11. Spoon the Mediterranean Tomato Sauce over each cod fillet.
12. Garnish with fresh chopped parsley and, if desired, fresh basil leaves.

Serve your Baked Cod with Mediterranean Tomato Sauce hot, with your choice of side dishes like couscous, rice, or steamed vegetables. Enjoy this flavorful and healthy fish dish!

Shrimp and Spinach Quiche

! Here's a recipe for Shrimp and Spinach Quiche:

.Ingredients:.

For the Quiche Filling:

- 1 9-inch pie crust (store-bought or homemade)

- 1/2 pound cooked shrimp, peeled and deveined

- 1 cup fresh spinach leaves, chopped

- 1/2 cup shredded Swiss cheese

- 4 large eggs

- 1 cup milk

- 1/2 teaspoon salt

- 1/4 teaspoon black pepper

- 1/4 teaspoon ground nutmeg

- 1/4 teaspoon paprika

- 1/4 teaspoon garlic powder

- 1/4 teaspoon onion powder

.Prepare the Quiche Crust:.

1. Preheat your oven to 375°F (190°C).
2. Place the pie crust in a 9-inch pie dish, crimping the edges if necessary. Prick the bottom of the crust with a fork to prevent it from puffing up during baking.
3. Pre-bake the pie crust in the preheated oven for about 10 minutes, or until it's set but not fully browned. Remove it from the oven and let it cool slightly.

.Prepare the Quiche Filling:.

4. In a medium-sized bowl, whisk together the eggs, milk, salt, black pepper, ground nutmeg, paprika, garlic powder, and onion powder until well combined.
5. Scatter the chopped fresh spinach leaves evenly over the pre-baked pie crust.
6. Arrange the cooked shrimp over the spinach.

7. Sprinkle the shredded Swiss cheese evenly over the
    shrimp and spinach.

.Assemble and Bake:.

8. Slowly pour the egg mixture over the shrimp,
    spinach, and cheese, ensuring that it's evenly
    distributed.
9. Place the quiche in the preheated oven and bake
    for 30-35 minutes, or until the quiche is set and the
    top is lightly golden brown.
10. Remove the quiche from the oven and let it cool for
    a few minutes before slicing and serving.

.Serve:.

11. Slice and serve your Shrimp and Spinach Quiche
    warm or at room temperature.

Enjoy your homemade Shrimp and Spinach Quiche as a
delicious and savory dish for brunch or a light dinner!

Tofu and Vegetable Kebabs

! Here's a recipe for Tofu and Vegetable Kebabs with Peanut Sauce:

.Ingredients:.

For the Tofu and Vegetable Kebabs:

- 14 ounces (about 1 block) extra-firm tofu, cut into cubes

- 1 red bell pepper, cut into chunks

- 1 yellow bell pepper, cut into chunks

- 1 zucchini, sliced into rounds

- 1 red onion, cut into chunks

- 8-10 wooden skewers, soaked in water for 30 minutes

For the Peanut Sauce:

- 1/4 cup peanut butter

- 2 tablespoons soy sauce

- 2 tablespoons rice vinegar

- 2 tablespoons maple syrup or honey

- 2 cloves garlic, minced

- 1 teaspoon grated fresh ginger

- 1/4 teaspoon red pepper flakes (adjust to taste)

- 2-3 tablespoons warm water (to thin the sauce)

- Chopped peanuts and chopped cilantro for garnish (optional)

.Instructions:.

.Prepare the Tofu and Vegetable Kebabs:.

1. In a bowl, combine the cubed tofu and your choice of vegetables (bell peppers, zucchini, and red onion).
2. Thread the tofu and vegetables onto the soaked wooden skewers, alternating between them.

.Make the Peanut Sauce:.

3. In a separate bowl, whisk together the peanut butter, soy sauce, rice vinegar, maple syrup (or honey), minced garlic, grated ginger, and red pepper flakes.
4. Add warm water to the peanut sauce, one tablespoon at a time, until you reach your desired consistency. The sauce should be smooth and pourable.

.Grill or Cook the Kebabs:.

5. Preheat your grill or grill pan to medium-high heat.
    If using a grill pan, lightly grease it.
6. Place the tofu and vegetable kebabs on the grill or
    grill pan and cook for about 3-4 minutes per side, or
    until they have grill marks and the tofu is heated
    through.

.Serve:.

7. Arrange the grilled tofu and vegetable kebabs on a
    serving platter.
8. Drizzle the peanut sauce over the kebabs.
9. Garnish with chopped peanuts and chopped
    cilantro, if desired.
10. Serve your Tofu and Vegetable Kebabs with Peanut
    Sauce hot, accompanied by rice or noodles if you
    like.

Enjoy this flavorful and protein-rich dish with the
creamy goodness of peanut sauce!

]

Grilled Mackerel with Citrus-Herb Marinade

! Here's a recipe for Grilled Mackerel with Citrus-Herb Marinade:

.Ingredients:.

For the Citrus-Herb Marinade:

- Zest and juice of 1 lemon

- Zest and juice of 1 orange

- 2 cloves garlic, minced

- 2 tablespoons fresh parsley, chopped

- 1 tablespoon fresh thyme leaves (or 1 teaspoon dried thyme)

- 1 tablespoon fresh rosemary leaves (or 1 teaspoon dried rosemary)

- 1/4 cup extra-virgin olive oil

- Salt and black pepper to taste

For the Grilled Mackerel:

- 4 mackerel fillets

- Salt and black pepper to taste

- Olive oil (for brushing the grill grates)

.Prepare the Citrus-Herb Marinade:.

1. In a bowl, combine the lemon zest, lemon juice, orange zest, orange juice, minced garlic, chopped fresh parsley, fresh thyme leaves (or dried thyme), fresh rosemary leaves (or dried rosemary), extra-virgin olive oil, salt, and black pepper.
2. Whisk the marinade ingredients until well combined.

.Marinate the Mackerel:.

3. Place the mackerel fillets in a shallow dish or a resealable plastic bag.
4. Pour the citrus-herb marinade over the mackerel fillets, ensuring they are well coated.
5. Seal the dish or bag and refrigerate for at least 30 minutes to allow the flavors to infuse the fish. You can marinate for longer for a more intense flavor.

.Preheat and Oil the Grill:.

6. Preheat your grill to medium-high heat. Brush the grill grates with olive oil to prevent sticking.

.Grill the Mackerel:.

7. Remove the mackerel fillets from the marinade and
   let any excess marinade drip off.
8. Season both sides of the mackerel fillets with salt
   and black pepper.
9. Place the mackerel fillets on the preheated grill and
   cook for about 3-4 minutes per side, or until they
   are opaque and easily flake with a fork. The cooking
   time may vary depending on the thickness of the
   fillets.

.Serve:.

10. Remove the grilled mackerel from the grill and
    transfer them to a serving platter.
11. Garnish with additional fresh herbs and citrus zest if
    desired.
12. Serve your Grilled Mackerel with Citrus-Herb
    Marinade hot, with your choice of side dishes like
    roasted vegetables or a fresh salad.

Enjoy the delicious and citrusy flavor of this grilled
mackerel dish!

Zucchini Noodles with Pesto

Here's a recipe for Zucchini Noodles with Pesto and Cherry Tomatoes, topped with Grilled Prawns:

.Ingredients:.

For the Zucchini Noodles:

- 4 medium zucchinis, spiralized into noodles

- Salt and black pepper to taste

- Olive oil for cooking

For the Pesto:

- 2 cups fresh basil leaves, packed

- 1/2 cup grated Parmesan cheese

- 1/2 cup pine nuts or walnuts

- 2 cloves garlic

- 1/2 cup extra-virgin olive oil

- Salt and black pepper to taste

- Juice of 1 lemon

For the Cherry Tomato Topping:

- 1 cup cherry tomatoes, halved

- 2 tablespoons olive oil

- Salt and black pepper to taste

For the Grilled Prawns:

- 1 pound large prawns or shrimp, peeled and deveined

- 2 tablespoons olive oil

- 2 cloves garlic, minced

- Salt and black pepper to taste

- Lemon wedges for serving (optional)

.Instructions:.

.Prepare the Pesto:.

1. In a food processor, combine the fresh basil, grated Parmesan cheese, pine nuts or walnuts, and garlic.
2. Pulse until the ingredients are finely chopped.
3. With the food processor running, slowly drizzle in the extra-virgin olive oil until the pesto reaches your desired consistency.
4. Add salt, black pepper, and lemon juice to taste. Adjust the seasoning as needed. Set the pesto aside.

.Grill the Prawns:.

5. In a bowl, combine the prawns or shrimp with olive oil, minced garlic, salt, and black pepper. Toss to coat evenly.

6. Preheat your grill or grill pan to medium-high heat.

7. Thread the marinated prawns onto skewers.

8. Grill the prawns for about 2-3 minutes per side, or until they turn pink and opaque. Remove them from the grill and set aside.

.Prepare the Cherry Tomato Topping:.

9. In a skillet, heat 2 tablespoons of olive oil over medium-high heat.

10. Add the halved cherry tomatoes and cook for about 2-3 minutes, or until they start to soften. Season with salt and black pepper. Remove from heat and set aside.

.Cook the Zucchini Noodles:.

11. In a large skillet, heat a bit of olive oil over medium heat.

12. Add the spiralized zucchini noodles and cook for about 2-3 minutes, tossing gently, until they are just heated through. Be careful not to overcook;

zucchini noodles should be tender but still slightly crisp.

.Assemble the Dish:.

13. Divide the cooked zucchini noodles among serving plates.

14. Spoon a generous amount of pesto over the noodles.

15. Top with the grilled prawns and the sautéed cherry tomatoes.

16. Garnish with lemon wedges if desired.

Serve your Zucchini Noodles with Pesto and Cherry Tomatoes, topped with Grilled Prawns, as a delicious and healthy seafood dish!

Seared Ahi Tuna Steaks

! Here's a recipe for Seared Ahi Tuna Steaks with Wasabi Sauce:

.Ingredients:.

For the Seared Ahi Tuna Steaks:

- 4 Ahi tuna steaks (about 6-8 ounces each)

- 2 tablespoons soy sauce

- 1 tablespoon sesame oil

- 1 teaspoon black sesame seeds (optional)

- Salt and black pepper to taste

- 2 tablespoons vegetable oil (for searing)

For the Wasabi Sauce:

- 2 tablespoons mayonnaise

- 1 tablespoon soy sauce

- 1-2 teaspoons wasabi paste (adjust to taste)

- 1 teaspoon honey or maple syrup

- 1 teaspoon rice vinegar

- 1 teaspoon fresh ginger, grated (optional)

.Instructions:.

.Prepare the Wasabi Sauce:.

1. In a small bowl, whisk together the mayonnaise, soy sauce, wasabi paste (start with 1 teaspoon and adjust for desired heat), honey or maple syrup, rice vinegar, and grated fresh ginger (if using). Taste and adjust the seasoning if needed. Set the sauce aside.

.Marinate and Sear the Ahi Tuna:.

2. In a shallow dish, combine the soy sauce, sesame oil, black sesame seeds (if using), salt, and black pepper.

3. Place the Ahi tuna steaks in the marinade, turning to coat them evenly. Allow the tuna to marinate for about 15-30 minutes in the refrigerator.

4. Heat the vegetable oil in a skillet or frying pan over high heat.

5. Remove the tuna steaks from the marinade and let any excess marinade drip off.

6. Sear the tuna steaks for about 1-2 minutes per side for rare to medium-rare, or longer if you prefer them more well-done. Keep in mind that Ahi tuna is typically enjoyed rare to medium-rare for the best flavor and texture.

.Serve:.

7. Remove the seared Ahi tuna steaks from the skillet and let them rest for a minute before slicing.

8. Slice the tuna steaks into thin strips.

9. Serve the Seared Ahi Tuna Steaks hot, drizzled with the prepared Wasabi Sauce.

Enjoy your Seared Ahi Tuna Steaks with Wasabi Sauce, a delightful combination of flavors and textures!

Coconut Curry Shrimp and Vegetables

! Here's a recipe for Coconut Curry Shrimp and Vegetables:

.Ingredients:.

For the Coconut Curry Sauce:

- 1 can (14 ounces) coconut milk

- 2 tablespoons red curry paste

- 2 tablespoons fish sauce (or soy sauce for a vegetarian version)

- 1 tablespoon brown sugar

- Juice of 1 lime

- 2 cloves garlic, minced

- 1 teaspoon fresh ginger, grated

- Salt and black pepper to taste

For the Shrimp and Vegetables:

- 1 pound large shrimp, peeled and deveined

- 2 tablespoons vegetable oil

- 1 onion, thinly sliced

- 1 red bell pepper, thinly sliced

- 1 yellow bell pepper, thinly sliced

- 1 zucchini, thinly sliced

- 1 cup broccoli florets

- Fresh cilantro leaves, for garnish

- Cooked rice or noodles, for serving

.Instructions:.

.Prepare the Coconut Curry Sauce:.

1. In a bowl, whisk together the coconut milk, red curry paste, fish sauce (or soy sauce), brown sugar, lime juice, minced garlic, grated ginger, salt, and black pepper. Set aside.

.Cook the Shrimp and Vegetables:.

2. In a large skillet or wok, heat the vegetable oil over medium-high heat.

3. Add the thinly sliced onion and sauté for about 2-3 minutes until it becomes translucent.

4. Add the thinly sliced red and yellow bell peppers, sliced zucchini, and broccoli florets to the skillet. Stir-fry for 4-5 minutes until the vegetables start to soften.

5. Push the vegetables to one side of the skillet and add the peeled and deveined shrimp to the other side. Cook the shrimp for about 2-3 minutes per side, or until they turn pink and opaque.

.Simmer with the Coconut Curry Sauce:.

6. Pour the prepared Coconut Curry Sauce over the cooked shrimp and vegetables in the skillet.

7. Stir to combine everything and allow it to simmer for an additional 2-3 minutes to heat the sauce and meld the flavors.

.Serve:.

8. Remove the Coconut Curry Shrimp and Vegetables from the heat.

9. Garnish with fresh cilantro leaves.

10. Serve hot over cooked rice or noodles.

Enjoy your Coconut Curry Shrimp and Vegetables, a flavorful and aromatic dish with a touch of Thai-inspired goodness!

Grilled Sardines with Mediterranean Salad:

! Here's a recipe for Grilled Sardines with Mediterranean Salad:

.Ingredients:.

For the Grilled Sardines:

- 8 fresh sardines, cleaned and gutted

- 2 tablespoons olive oil

- 2 cloves garlic, minced

- 1 lemon, sliced into rounds

- Salt and black pepper to taste

- Fresh parsley, chopped, for garnish (optional)

For the Mediterranean Salad:

- 2 cups cherry tomatoes, halved

- 1 cucumber, diced

- 1 red onion, thinly sliced

- 1/2 cup Kalamata olives, pitted

- 1/2 cup feta cheese, crumbled

- Fresh basil leaves, torn

- Salt and black pepper to taste

- Extra-virgin olive oil and red wine vinegar (for
dressing)

.Instructions:.

.Prepare the Grilled Sardines:.

1.   Preheat your grill to medium-high heat.

2.   In a small bowl, mix the olive oil and minced garlic.

3.   Brush the sardines with the garlic-infused olive oil

     on both sides, and season them with salt and black

     pepper.

4.   Place a lemon slice inside each sardine cavity.

5.   Grill the sardines for about 3-4 minutes per side, or

     until they are cooked through and have grill marks.

     Be gentle when flipping to prevent them from

     falling apart.

.Prepare the Mediterranean Salad:.

6.   In a large bowl, combine the halved cherry

     tomatoes, diced cucumber, thinly sliced red onion,

     pitted Kalamata olives, crumbled feta cheese, and

     torn fresh basil leaves.

7. Season the salad with salt and black pepper to taste.

8. Drizzle extra-virgin olive oil and red wine vinegar over the salad, adjusting to your preferred taste.

9. Toss the salad to coat the ingredients evenly with the dressing.

.Serve:.

10. Arrange the grilled sardines on a serving platter.

11. Spoon the Mediterranean Salad alongside the sardines.

12. Garnish with fresh chopped parsley, if desired.

Serve your Grilled Sardines with Mediterranean Salad for a delicious and nutritious meal inspired by Mediterranean flavors. Enjoy!.

Teriyaki Glazed Grilled Tofu

! Here's a recipe for Teriyaki Glazed Grilled Tofu:

.Ingredients:.

For the Teriyaki Marinade and Glaze:

- 1/2 cup soy sauce

- 1/4 cup water

- 3 tablespoons brown sugar

- 2 tablespoons rice vinegar

- 2 cloves garlic, minced

- 1 teaspoon fresh ginger, grated

- 1 tablespoon cornstarch (for thickening)

For the Grilled Tofu:

- 1 block (about 14 ounces) extra-firm tofu

- 2 tablespoons vegetable oil (for brushing)

- Sesame seeds and chopped green onions for garnish (optional)

.Instructions:.

.Prepare the Teriyaki Marinade and Glaze:.

1. In a small saucepan, combine the soy sauce, water, brown sugar, rice vinegar, minced garlic, and grated ginger.

2. In a separate small bowl, whisk the cornstarch with a couple of tablespoons of water until it forms a smooth slurry.

3. Heat the saucepan with the marinade over medium heat until it comes to a simmer.

4. Stir in the cornstarch slurry into the simmering marinade. Continue to cook and stir until the sauce thickens and becomes glossy. Remove it from heat. This is your teriyaki glaze.

.Prepare the Tofu:.

5. Press the tofu to remove excess moisture. You can use a tofu press or wrap the tofu block in paper towels and place a heavy object on top. Let it press for about 15-20 minutes.

6. Slice the pressed tofu into 1/2-inch thick slabs or cubes, depending on your preference.

7. Brush the tofu slabs or cubes with vegetable oil to prevent sticking to the grill.

.Grill the Tofu:.

8. Preheat your grill to medium-high heat. If using a grill pan, heat it on the stovetop.

9. Place the tofu slabs or cubes on the grill and cook for about 3-4 minutes on each side, or until grill marks form and the tofu is heated through.

.Glaze the Tofu:.

10. Brush the teriyaki glaze generously over the grilled tofu while it's still on the grill.
11. Continue grilling for another 1-2 minutes on each side, brushing with more glaze, until the tofu has absorbed the flavors and has a nice caramelized coating.

.Serve:.

12. Remove the glazed grilled tofu from the grill.
13. Garnish with sesame seeds and chopped green onions if desired.

Serve your Teriyaki Glazed Grilled Tofu hot, either on its own, with rice, or in a stir-fry. Enjoy the sweet and savory flavors of this tofu dish!

Smoked Trout and Cucumber Tea Sandwiches

! Here's a recipe for Smoked Trout and Cucumber Tea Sandwiches:

.Ingredients:.

- 8 slices of your favorite bread (white, whole wheat, or rye)

- 4 ounces smoked trout (or smoked salmon)

- 1 small cucumber, thinly sliced

- 4 tablespoons cream cheese, softened

- 1-2 tablespoons fresh dill, chopped

- 1 lemon, zested

- Salt and black pepper to taste

.Instructions:.

.Prepare the Spread:.

1. In a small bowl, mix the softened cream cheese, chopped fresh dill, lemon zest, salt, and black pepper. This will be your spread for the sandwiches.

.Assemble the Tea Sandwiches:.

2. Lay out the slices of bread.
3. Spread a generous layer of the dill and lemon cream cheese mixture onto one side of each slice of bread.
4. Lay the thinly sliced cucumber on half of the bread slices, ensuring they cover the cream cheese mixture.

5. Place the smoked trout (or smoked salmon) on top of the cucumber slices.

6. Top with the remaining slices of bread, cream cheese side down, to create sandwiches.

.Cut and Serve:.

7. Using a sharp knife, remove the crusts from each sandwich.

8. Cut each sandwich into bite-sized pieces or rectangles to create tea sandwiches.

9. Arrange the Smoked Trout and Cucumber Tea Sandwiches on a serving platter.

.Serve:.

10. Serve your tea sandwiches immediately for a delightful and elegant snack or as part of a tea-time spread.

Enjoy these delicate and flavorful Smoked Trout and Cucumber Tea Sandwiches as a delightful treat for a tea party or a light, sophisticated snack!

Quinoa and Black Bean Stuffed Bell Peppers

! Here's a recipe for Quinoa and Black Bean Stuffed Bell Peppers with Shrimp:

.Ingredients:.

For the Stuffed Bell Peppers:

- 4 large bell peppers (any color), tops removed and seeds removed

- 1 cup quinoa, rinsed and cooked according to package instructions

- 1 can (15 ounces) black beans, drained and rinsed

- 1 cup corn kernels (fresh, frozen, or canned)

- 1 cup diced tomatoes (canned or fresh)

- 1 teaspoon chili powder

- 1/2 teaspoon cumin

- Salt and black pepper to taste

- 1 cup shredded cheddar cheese (or your favorite cheese)

For the Shrimp:

- 1 pound large shrimp, peeled and deveined

- 2 tablespoons olive oil

- 2 cloves garlic, minced

- 1 teaspoon paprika

- Salt and black pepper to taste

- Fresh cilantro leaves for garnish (optional)

.Instructions:.

.Prepare the Stuffed Bell Peppers:.

1. Preheat your oven to 375°F (190°C).
2. In a large mixing bowl, combine the cooked quinoa, black beans, corn kernels, diced tomatoes, chili powder, cumin, salt, and black pepper. Mix well.
3. Carefully stuff each bell pepper with the quinoa and black bean mixture, pressing it down gently.
4. Sprinkle shredded cheese over the tops of the stuffed peppers.
5. Place the stuffed bell peppers in a baking dish and cover with aluminum foil.
6. Bake in the preheated oven for 25-30 minutes, or until the peppers are tender and the cheese is melted and bubbly.

.Prepare the Shrimp:.

7. While the peppers are baking, prepare the shrimp.

8. In a large skillet, heat the olive oil over medium-high heat.

9. Add the minced garlic and cook for about 30 seconds until fragrant.

10. Season the shrimp with paprika, salt, and black pepper.

11. Add the seasoned shrimp to the skillet and cook for 2-3 minutes per side, or until they turn pink and opaque.

.Serve:.

12. Remove the stuffed bell peppers from the oven.

13. Place the cooked shrimp on top of each stuffed pepper.

14. Garnish with fresh cilantro leaves if desired.

Serve your Quinoa and Black Bean Stuffed Bell Peppers with Shrimp as a flavorful and nutritious meal. Enjoy!

Lemon Garlic Butter Shrimp

! Here's a recipe for Lemon Garlic Butter Shrimp and Asparagus:

.Ingredients:.

- 1 pound large shrimp, peeled and deveined

- 1 bunch fresh asparagus, trimmed and cut into 2-inch pieces

- 4 cloves garlic, minced

- 2 tablespoons olive oil

- 2 tablespoons unsalted butter

- Zest and juice of 1 lemon

- Salt and black pepper to taste

- Fresh parsley or dill, chopped, for garnish (optional)

.Instructions:.

.Prepare the Shrimp and Asparagus:.

1.   Season the peeled and deveined shrimp with a pinch of salt and black pepper. Set aside.

2.   In a large skillet or frying pan, heat the olive oil over medium-high heat.

3. Add the minced garlic and sauté for about 30
    seconds until fragrant, but do not let it brown.

4. Add the trimmed asparagus pieces to the skillet and
    sauté for about 3-4 minutes, or until they start to
    become tender.

.Cook the Shrimp:.

5. Push the asparagus to one side of the skillet and
    add the butter to the other side.

6. Add the seasoned shrimp to the skillet.

7. Cook the shrimp for about 2-3 minutes per side, or
    until they turn pink and opaque.

.Add Lemon Flavor:.

8. Once the shrimp are cooked, add the lemon zest
    and lemon juice to the skillet. Stir to combine,
    allowing the flavors to meld for another minute.

.Garnish and Serve:.

9. Garnish with freshly chopped parsley or dill if
    desired.

10. Serve your Lemon Garlic Butter Shrimp and
    Asparagus hot as a delicious and flavorful meal.

This dish is perfect for a quick and satisfying dinner!

Avocado and Tuna Salad Wraps

! Here's a recipe for Avocado and Tuna Salad Wraps:

.Ingredients:.

For the Tuna Salad:

- 2 cans (5 ounces each) of tuna in water, drained

- 1 ripe avocado, diced

- 1/4 cup red onion, finely chopped

- 1/4 cup celery, finely chopped

- 1/4 cup mayonnaise (adjust to your preference)

- 1 tablespoon fresh lemon juice

- Salt and black pepper to taste

- Optional: 1/2 teaspoon Dijon mustard for extra flavor

For the Wraps:

- Large lettuce leaves (such as Romaine or iceberg) or your favorite tortillas/wraps

- Sliced cucumber

- Sliced tomato

- Sliced red bell pepper

- Sliced carrot

- Fresh spinach or arugula leaves

- Sliced avocado

- Lemon wedges for serving (optional)

.Instructions:.

.Prepare the Tuna Salad:.

1. In a mixing bowl, combine the drained tuna, diced avocado, chopped red onion, chopped celery, mayonnaise, fresh lemon juice, and Dijon mustard (if using).
2. Gently fold the ingredients together until well combined.
3. Season the tuna salad with salt and black pepper to taste. Adjust the seasoning and lemon juice to your preference.

.Assemble the Wraps:.

4. Lay out your choice of large lettuce leaves or tortillas/wraps on a clean surface.

5. Place a generous spoonful of the tuna salad mixture onto each lettuce leaf or tortilla.

6. Add slices of cucumber, tomato, red bell pepper, carrot, avocado, and fresh spinach or arugula on top of the tuna salad.

.Wrap and Serve:.

7. If using lettuce leaves, fold the sides over the filling and roll up tightly, securing with a toothpick if needed. If using tortillas, fold in the sides and roll them up.

8. Serve your Avocado and Tuna Salad Wraps with lemon wedges for an extra zesty touch, if desired.

Enjoy these refreshing and healthy wraps as a light and satisfying meal or snack!

Creamy Spinach and Artichoke

! Here's a recipe for Creamy Spinach and Artichoke Stuffed Portobello Mushrooms with Shrimp:

.Ingredients:.

For the Stuffed Portobello Mushrooms:

- 4 large Portobello mushrooms, stems removed and cleaned

- 1 tablespoon olive oil

- 2 cloves garlic, minced

- 1/2 cup onion, finely chopped

- 1 cup fresh spinach, chopped

- 1/2 cup canned artichoke hearts, chopped

- 1/2 cup cream cheese

- 1/4 cup grated Parmesan cheese

- Salt and black pepper to taste

For the Shrimp:

- 1 pound large shrimp, peeled and deveined

- 1 tablespoon olive oil

- 2 cloves garlic, minced

- 1 teaspoon paprika

- Salt and black pepper to taste

- Lemon wedges for serving (optional)

.Prepare the Stuffed Portobello Mushrooms:.

1. Preheat your oven to 375°F (190°C).
2. Place the cleaned Portobello mushrooms on a baking sheet, cap side down. Drizzle olive oil over them and season with salt and black pepper.
3. Roast the mushrooms in the preheated oven for about 10 minutes to remove excess moisture. Remove and set aside.
4. In a skillet, heat olive oil over medium heat. Add minced garlic and chopped onion, and sauté until the onion becomes translucent.
5. Add chopped spinach and sauté until it wilts.
6. Stir in the chopped artichoke hearts and cook for an additional 2-3 minutes.
7. Reduce the heat to low, then add cream cheese and grated Parmesan cheese. Stir until the cheeses melt and the mixture becomes creamy. Season with salt and black pepper to taste.
8. Fill each roasted Portobello mushroom cap with the creamy spinach and artichoke mixture.

.Prepare the Shrimp:.

9. In a separate skillet, heat olive oil over medium-high heat.

10. Add minced garlic and cook for about 30 seconds until fragrant.

11. Season the peeled and deveined shrimp with paprika, salt, and black pepper.

12. Add the seasoned shrimp to the skillet and cook for about 2-3 minutes per side, or until they turn pink and opaque.

.Serve:.

13. Place the cooked shrimp on top of the stuffed Portobello mushrooms.

14. Optionally, squeeze fresh lemon juice over the shrimp for added flavor.

15. Serve your Creamy Spinach and Artichoke Stuffed Portobello Mushrooms with Shrimp as a delicious and elegant meal.

Enjoy this flavorful and satisfying dish!

Grilled Mahi-Mahi with Pineapple Salsa

! Here's a recipe for Grilled Mahi-Mahi with Pineapple Salsa:

.Ingredients:.

For the Grilled Mahi-Mahi:

- 4 Mahi-Mahi fillets (about 6-8 ounces each)

- 2 tablespoons olive oil

- 2 cloves garlic, minced

- 1 teaspoon paprika

- 1 teaspoon cumin

- 1/2 teaspoon chili powder (adjust to taste)

- Salt and black pepper to taste

- Lemon wedges for serving (optional)

For the Pineapple Salsa:

- 2 cups fresh pineapple, diced

- 1/2 red onion, finely chopped

- 1/2 red bell pepper, diced

- 1/4 cup fresh cilantro, chopped

- 1 jalapeño pepper, seeded and finely chopped (adjust to taste)

- Juice of 1 lime

- Salt and black pepper to taste

.Instructions:.

.Prepare the Pineapple Salsa:.

1. In a mixing bowl, combine the diced fresh pineapple, finely chopped red onion, diced red bell pepper, chopped fresh cilantro, and finely chopped jalapeño pepper.
2. Squeeze the juice of one lime over the mixture and gently toss to combine.
3. Season the pineapple salsa with salt and black pepper to taste. Adjust the seasoning and add more lime juice if desired. Refrigerate the salsa until you're ready to serve.

.Prepare the Grilled Mahi-Mahi:.

4. In a small bowl, mix the olive oil, minced garlic, paprika, cumin, chili powder, salt, and black pepper to create a marinade.

5. Brush the Mahi-Mahi fillets with the marinade on
    both sides. Allow them to marinate for about 15-20
    minutes at room temperature.

6. Preheat your grill to medium-high heat. Make sure
    the grill grates are clean and lightly oiled to prevent
    sticking.

7. Grill the Mahi-Mahi fillets for about 3-4 minutes per
    side, or until they are opaque and easily flake with a
    fork. Cooking time may vary depending on the
    thickness of the fillets.

.Serve:.

8. Remove the grilled Mahi-Mahi from the grill.

9. Serve the grilled Mahi-Mahi fillets hot, topped with
    a generous spoonful of the pineapple salsa.

10. Optionally, garnish with fresh cilantro and offer
    lemon wedges for an extra zesty touch.

Enjoy your Grilled Mahi-Mahi with Pineapple Salsa for a
tropical and flavorful seafood dish!

Tofu and Vegetable Stir-Fry

! Here's a recipe for Tofu and Vegetable Stir-Fry with Soy-Ginger Sauce:

.Ingredients:.

For the Stir-Fry:

- 1 block (about 14 ounces) extra-firm tofu, pressed and cubed

- 2 cups mixed vegetables (broccoli florets, bell peppers, snap peas, carrots, etc.), sliced or chopped

- 2 tablespoons vegetable oil for stir-frying

- Salt and black pepper to taste

For the Soy-Ginger Sauce:

- 1/4 cup soy sauce

- 2 tablespoons rice vinegar

- 2 tablespoons honey or maple syrup

- 1 tablespoon fresh ginger, minced

- 2 cloves garlic, minced

- 1 teaspoon cornstarch mixed with 1 tablespoon cold water (for thickening)

.Prepare the Soy-Ginger Sauce:.

1. In a small bowl, whisk together the soy sauce, rice vinegar, honey or maple syrup, minced fresh ginger, and minced garlic.
2. In a separate small bowl, mix the cornstarch with cold water until it forms a smooth slurry.
3. Heat the soy sauce mixture in a saucepan over medium heat. Once it begins to simmer, stir in the cornstarch slurry.
4. Continue to simmer, stirring constantly, until the sauce thickens and becomes glossy. Remove it from heat. This is your soy-ginger sauce.

.Prepare the Tofu and Vegetables:.

5. In a large skillet or wok, heat the vegetable oil over medium-high heat.
6. Add the cubed tofu to the hot skillet and stir-fry for about 4-5 minutes until it becomes golden and slightly crispy on the outside. Remove the tofu from the skillet and set it aside.
7. In the same skillet, add a bit more oil if needed, and then add the mixed vegetables. Stir-fry for about 3-

4 minutes, or until they are tender-crisp. Season with salt and black pepper to taste.

.Combine and Serve:.

8. Return the cooked tofu to the skillet with the stir-fried vegetables.

9. Pour the soy-ginger sauce over the tofu and vegetables.

10. Stir-fry for an additional 2-3 minutes, or until everything is well coated with the sauce and heated through.

11. Serve your Tofu and Vegetable Stir-Fry hot, over cooked rice or noodles if desired.

Enjoy your Tofu and Vegetable Stir-Fry with Soy-Ginger Sauce, a delicious and satisfying plant-based meal!

Grilled Swordfish with Mango Salsa

! Here's a recipe for Grilled Swordfish with Mango Salsa:

.Ingredients:.

For the Grilled Swordfish:

- 4 swordfish steaks (about 6-8 ounces each)

- 2 tablespoons olive oil

- 2 cloves garlic, minced

- 1 teaspoon paprika

- 1/2 teaspoon dried oregano

- Salt and black pepper to taste

- Lemon wedges for serving (optional)

For the Mango Salsa:

- 2 ripe mangoes, peeled, pitted, and diced

- 1/2 red onion, finely chopped

- 1 red bell pepper, diced

- 1 jalapeño pepper, seeded and finely chopped (adjust to taste)

- 1/4 cup fresh cilantro, chopped

- Juice of 1 lime

- Salt and black pepper to taste

.Instructions:.

.Prepare the Grilled Swordfish:.

1. In a small bowl, mix together olive oil, minced garlic, paprika, dried oregano, salt, and black pepper.

2. Brush the swordfish steaks on both sides with the
    olive oil mixture.

3. Preheat your grill to medium-high heat. Make sure
    the grill grates are clean and lightly oiled.

4. Grill the swordfish steaks for about 4-5 minutes per
    side, or until they are cooked through and have grill
    marks. Cooking time may vary depending on the
    thickness of the steaks.

.Prepare the Mango Salsa:.

5. While the swordfish is grilling, prepare the mango
    salsa. In a mixing bowl, combine the diced mangoes,
    finely chopped red onion, diced red bell pepper,
    finely chopped jalapeño pepper, chopped fresh
    cilantro, and the juice of one lime.

6. Season the salsa with salt and black pepper to taste.
    Adjust the seasoning and lime juice according to
    your preference.

.Serve:.

7. Remove the grilled swordfish from the grill and let it
    rest for a minute.

8. Serve each swordfish steak hot, topped with a
    generous spoonful of the mango salsa.

9. Optionally, offer lemon wedges for squeezing over the grilled swordfish for added zest.

Enjoy your Grilled Swordfish with Mango Salsa, a delicious and vibrant dish!

Seafood Paella

! Here's a recipe for Seafood Paella:

.Ingredients:.

- 1 1/2 cups Arborio rice

- 1 pound mixed seafood (shrimp, mussels, squid, and/or clams)

- 1/2 cup diced onion

- 1/2 cup diced bell pepper (red or yellow)

- 1/2 cup diced tomatoes

- 3 cloves garlic, minced

- 4 cups seafood or vegetable broth

- 1/2 teaspoon saffron threads (optional for color and flavor)

- 1 teaspoon smoked paprika

- 1/2 teaspoon paprika

- 1/2 teaspoon turmeric (for color)

- 1/4 cup dry white wine (optional)

- 2 tablespoons olive oil

- Salt and black pepper to taste

- Fresh parsley or lemon wedges for garnish

.Instructions:.

.Prepare the Saffron Infusion:.

1. In a small bowl, crush the saffron threads slightly, and then soak them in a couple of tablespoons of hot water. Let it steep to release the flavor and color.

.Cook the Seafood:.

2. In a large paella pan or a wide skillet, heat the olive oil over medium-high heat.
3. Add the mixed seafood to the hot pan and cook for about 2-3 minutes, or until they start to turn opaque. Remove them from the pan and set aside.

.Sauté the Aromatics:.

4. In the same pan, add diced onion, diced bell pepper, and minced garlic. Sauté for about 3-4 minutes until the vegetables soften.

.Add the Rice and Spices:.

5. Stir in the Arborio rice, smoked paprika, paprika, and turmeric. Toast the rice for 2-3 minutes, stirring frequently.
6. Pour in the white wine (if using) and let it cook for a minute or two until it mostly evaporates.

.Simmer with Broth and Saffron:.

7. Add the diced tomatoes to the rice mixture and cook for another 2 minutes.
8. Pour the saffron infusion over the rice.
9. Start adding the seafood or vegetable broth, one cup at a time, allowing the rice to absorb the liquid before adding more. Stir occasionally.

.Add Seafood Back In:.

10. Once the rice is almost tender and the liquid is mostly absorbed (about 15-20 minutes), return the cooked seafood to the pan. Place them evenly on top of the rice.

11. Continue to cook for another 5-7 minutes, or until
    the rice is fully cooked, and the seafood is heated
    through.

.Finish and Serve:.

12. Season the paella with salt and black pepper to
    taste.

13. Remove the paella from heat and let it rest for a
    few minutes.

14. Garnish with fresh parsley or lemon wedges before
    serving.

Serve your Seafood Paella hot, straight from the pan,
for a delightful Spanish-inspired dish!

Smoked Salmon and Cream Cheese Bagels

! Here's a classic recipe for Smoked Salmon and Cream
Cheese Bagels:

.Ingredients:.

- 4 bagels, sliced and toasted

- 4 ounces smoked salmon

- 4 ounces cream cheese, at room temperature

- Red onion, thinly sliced

- Capers

- Fresh dill sprigs

- Lemon wedges

- Salt and black pepper to taste

.Instructions:.

.Prepare the Bagels:.

1. Slice the bagels in half and toast them to your desired level of crispness.

.Assemble the Bagels:.

2. Spread a generous layer of cream cheese on each half of the toasted bagels.
3. Lay slices of smoked salmon on the bottom half of each bagel.
4. Top the smoked salmon with thinly sliced red onion and capers, adjusting the amount to your taste.
5. Add a sprig of fresh dill on top for extra flavor and garnish.

6.   Season with a pinch of salt and black pepper if
     desired.

.Serve:.

7.   Squeeze fresh lemon juice over the assembled
     bagels or serve them with lemon wedges on the
     side.
8.   Place the top half of the bagels over the salmon and
     other toppings to create a sandwich.
9.   Serve your Smoked Salmon and Cream Cheese
     Bagels immediately, and enjoy this classic and
     delicious combination!

This makes for a perfect breakfast, brunch, or even a
quick and satisfying snack.

Baked Halibut with Herbed Breadcrumbs

! Here's a recipe for Baked Halibut with Herbed
Breadcrumbs:

.Ingredients:.

For the Herbed Breadcrumbs:

- 1 cup fresh breadcrumbs (from day-old bread)

- 2 tablespoons fresh parsley, chopped

- 1 tablespoon fresh dill, chopped

- 1 clove garlic, minced

- Zest of 1 lemon

- 2 tablespoons olive oil

- Salt and black pepper to taste

For the Halibut:

- 4 halibut fillets (about 6 ounces each)

- 2 tablespoons olive oil

- Salt and black pepper to taste

- Lemon wedges for serving (optional)

.Instructions:.

.Prepare the Herbed Breadcrumbs:.

1.   In a mixing bowl, combine the fresh breadcrumbs, chopped fresh parsley, chopped fresh dill, minced garlic, lemon zest, olive oil, salt, and black pepper.

2.   Mix the ingredients together until the breadcrumbs are coated with the herbs and oil.

.Prepare the Halibut:.

3. Preheat your oven to 375°F (190°C). Line a baking
    sheet with parchment paper or lightly grease it.
4. Place the halibut fillets on the prepared baking
    sheet.
5. Brush the halibut fillets with olive oil and season
    them with salt and black pepper.

.Top with Herbed Breadcrumbs:.

6. Spoon the herbed breadcrumb mixture evenly over
    the top of each halibut fillet, pressing it down
    slightly to adhere.

.Bake the Halibut:.

7. Bake the halibut in the preheated oven for about
    12-15 minutes, or until the fish is cooked through
    and the breadcrumbs are golden brown and crispy.

.Serve:.

8. Remove the baked halibut from the oven.
9. Serve your Baked Halibut with Herbed Breadcrumbs
    hot, garnished with lemon wedges if desired.

Enjoy this flavorful and easy-to-make dish that's perfect
for a weeknight dinner or a special occasion!

Cilantro-Lime Grilled Shrimp Tacos

! Here's a recipe for Cilantro-Lime Grilled Shrimp Tacos:

.Ingredients:.

For the Grilled Shrimp:

- 1 pound large shrimp, peeled and deveined

- 2 cloves garlic, minced

- Zest and juice of 2 limes

- 2 tablespoons fresh cilantro, chopped

- 2 tablespoons olive oil

- Salt and black pepper to taste

- Taco seasoning (optional for extra flavor)

For the Cilantro-Lime Crema:

- 1/2 cup sour cream or Greek yogurt

- 2 tablespoons fresh cilantro, chopped

- Zest and juice of 1 lime

- Salt and black pepper to taste

For Assembling Tacos:

- 8 small flour or corn tortillas

- Shredded lettuce or cabbage

- Sliced avocado or guacamole

- Sliced red onion

- Sliced jalapeño (optional for heat)

- Lime wedges for serving

- Additional fresh cilantro for garnish

.Instructions:.

.Marinate and Grill the Shrimp:.

1. In a mixing bowl, combine the peeled and deveined shrimp with minced garlic, lime zest, lime juice, chopped cilantro, olive oil, salt, black pepper, and taco seasoning (if using). Toss to coat the shrimp evenly.

2. Thread the marinated shrimp onto skewers (if using wooden skewers, soak them in water for 30 minutes before threading).

3. Preheat your grill to medium-high heat. Make sure the grill grates are clean and lightly oiled.

4. Grill the shrimp skewers for about 2-3 minutes per side, or until they turn pink and slightly charred. Be

careful not to overcook them as shrimp can become tough.

.Prepare the Cilantro-Lime Crema:.

5. In a small bowl, mix together sour cream or Greek yogurt, chopped cilantro, lime zest, lime juice, salt, and black pepper. This is your cilantro-lime crema.

.Assemble the Tacos:.

6. Warm the tortillas on the grill or in a skillet for a minute or two.

7. Spread a spoonful of the cilantro-lime crema on each tortilla.

8. Place a portion of shredded lettuce or cabbage on top of the crema.

9. Add grilled shrimp, sliced avocado or guacamole, sliced red onion, and sliced jalapeño if desired.

10. Garnish with fresh cilantro leaves and serve with lime wedges for squeezing over the tacos.

11. Serve your Cilantro-Lime Grilled Shrimp Tacos hot and enjoy!

These tacos are bursting with fresh and zesty flavors, making them perfect for a delicious meal.

Mediterranean Tuna Salad

! Here's a recipe for Mediterranean Tuna Salad:

.Ingredients:.

- 2 cans (5 ounces each) of tuna in water, drained

- 1/2 cucumber, diced

- 1/2 red onion, finely chopped

- 1/2 cup cherry tomatoes, halved

- 1/2 cup Kalamata olives, pitted and sliced

- 1/4 cup fresh parsley, chopped

- 1/4 cup fresh basil leaves, torn

- 1/4 cup feta cheese, crumbled

- 2 tablespoons extra-virgin olive oil

- Juice of 1 lemon

- Salt and black pepper to taste

- Optional: 1/2 teaspoon dried oregano for extra flavor

.Instructions:.

1. In a large mixing bowl, flake the drained tuna with a
   fork to break it into smaller pieces.

2. Add diced cucumber, finely chopped red onion, halved cherry tomatoes, sliced Kalamata olives, chopped fresh parsley, torn fresh basil leaves, and crumbled feta cheese to the tuna.

3. Drizzle extra-virgin olive oil and the juice of one lemon over the salad.

4. If desired, sprinkle dried oregano over the salad for extra Mediterranean flavor.

5. Season the salad with salt and black pepper to taste.

6. Toss all the ingredients together until they are well combined.

7. Taste and adjust the seasoning, olive oil, or lemon juice according to your preference.

8. Refrigerate the Mediterranean Tuna Salad for at least 30 minutes before serving to allow the flavors to meld.

9. Serve the chilled salad on its own, with a side of crusty bread, or over a bed of fresh greens for a refreshing and healthy meal.

Enjoy your Mediterranean Tuna Salad, packed with Mediterranean-inspired flavors!

CONCLUTION

A pescatarian diet can be quite healthy.

What's more, it lets you avoid some of the ethical and environmental issues related to diets that include meat.

Additionally, this way of eating provides more flexibility and some additional nutrition compared to a standard vegetarian diet.

Overall, eating a plant-based diet with some seafood is a healthy choice.

www.ingramcontent.com/pod-product-compliance
Lightning Source LLC
Chambersburg PA
CBHW070940260726

48661CB00003B/1051